Integrating Psychotherapy and Pharmacotherapy

JARVIS

Integrating Psychotherapy and Pharmacotherapy

Dissolving the Mind-Brain Barrier

Bernard D. Beitman, M.D.

Barton J. Blinder, M.D., Ph.D.

Michael E. Thase, M.D.

Michelle Riba, M.D.

Debra L. Safer, M.D.

W·W·NORTON

NEW YORK · LONDON

For information about permission to reproduce
selections from this book, write to
Permissions, W. W. Norton & Company, Inc.
500 Fifth Avenue, New York, NY 10110

Composition and book design by Ecomlinks, Inc.
Manufacturing by Haddon Craftsman
Production Manager: Leeann Graham

Library of Congress Cataloging-in-Publication Data
Integrating psychotherapy and pharmacotherapy: dissolving the mind-brain barrier/
Bernard D. Beitman.
    p.   cm.
"A Norton professional book."
ISBN 0-393-70403-3 (pbk)
1. Mental illness—Chemotherapy. 2. Psychopharmacology 3. Psychotropic drugs.
4. Psychotherapy. 5. Combined modality therapy. I. Bernard D. Beitman.
[DNLM: 1. Mental Disorders—drug therapy. 2. Psychotherapy—methods. 3. Combined
Modality Therapy 4. Psychopharmacology. 5. Psychophysiology. WM 402 I611 2003]
RC480 .I456   2003
616.89'18—dc21   2002038060

W. W. Norton & Company, Inc., 500 Fifth Avenue, New York, NY 10110
www.wwnorton.com
W. W. Norton & Company, Ltd., Castle House, 75/76 Wells Street, London W1T 3QT

Contents

List of Authors vii

Preface ix

Introduction by Bernard D. Beitman, M.D. xv

Flow Chart for a Ten-Session Seminar Series xxi

PART I: ISSUES, VIGNETTES, AND COMMENTARY

Section 1. Research in Combined Treatments 3

Section 2. Pharmacotherapy During Psychotherapy 13

Section 3. Psychotherapy During Pharmacotherapy 35

Section 4. A Physician, a Nonmedical Psychotherapist, and
a Patient: The Pharmacotherapy-Psychotherapy
Triangle 73

Section 5. The Sequencing Problem (Using Panic Disorder . . . 85
as an Example)

Section 6. Briefly Toward a Neurobiology of Psychotherapy . . 105

PART II: RESEARCH PERSPECTIVES, SPLIT TREATMENT, AND PSYCHODYNAMIC NEUROBIOLOGY

Conceptual and Empirical Basis for Integrating Psychotherapy
and Pharmacotherapy
by Michael E. Thase, M.D. 111

The Challenges of Split Treatment
    by Michelle B. Riba, M.D. and Richard Balon, M.D. . 141
Psychodynamic Neurobiology
    by Barton J. Blinder, M.D., Ph.D. 161

    References 181
    Index 213

List of Authors

Richard Balon, M.D. is Professor of Psychiatry at the Department of Psychiatry and Behavioral Neurosciences, Wayne State University, Detroit, MI.

Bernard D. Beitman, M.D. is Professor and Chairman of the Department of Psychiatry at the University of Missouri-Columbia and a member of the Committee on Psychotherapy by Psychiatrists of the American Psychiatric Association.

Michael E. Thase, M.D. is Professor of Psychiatry, Department of Psychiatry, University of Pittsburgh Medical Center, Western Psychiatric Institute and Clinic.

Barton J. Blinder, M.D., Ph.D. is Clinical Professor and Director of Eating Disorder Research, Department of Psychiatry and Human Behavior, College of Medicine, University of California, Irvine.

Michelle Riba, M.D. is Clinical Professor of Psychiatry, Associate Chair for Education and Academic Affairs, Department of Psychiatry, University of Michigan.

Debra L. Safer, M.D. is Associate Director of Residency Training and Assistant Clinical Professor, Department of Psychiatry and Behavioral Sciences, Stanford University School of Medicine.

Preface

In an attempt to sharpen perspectives on the common factors in psychotherapy, in 1981 I published a paper titled *Pharmacotherapy as an intervention during the stages of psychotherapy*. The paper suggested that medications, in addition to their direct pharmacological actions, could function as another psychotherapeutic intervention. The prescription of medications could influence the development of the working alliance, highlight maladaptive patterns, evoke key dynamic issues involving resistance, transference and countertransference, as well as assist in the initiation and maintenance of change.

Spurred by the seminal work of Gerry Klerman and Myrna Weissman, researchers were beginning to study the combination of pharmacotherapy and psychotherapy in various psychiatric disorders. With Gerry's help, I organized a conference at the University of Washington in 1983 dedicated to gathering together the various researchers in this growing area. Two books edited by Gerry and me on this subject followed in 1984 and 1991.

Because of these efforts in studying combined treatment I was invited to join the American Psychiatric Association's Commission on Psychotherapy by Psychiatrists (COPP) chaired by Drew Clemens and later Jerry Kay. Among our several clear missions was the task to delineate more sharply the importance and understanding of combined treatment. At the same time, working with Dongmei Yue, I was attempting to develop a psychotherapy training program suitable for psychiatric residents and others that would be time efficient, research based and outcome-measured. That program was published as *Learning Psychotherapy* (1999) also by Norton, and has gained use by many psychiatric residency training programs. Its case vignette-based active learning has been a key factor in its success. Concurrently with the development of the psychotherapy program, I continued to collect case vignette that could serve as the basis for a module on integrating psychotherapy and pharmacotherapy. Part I of this book is the product of that effort.

Many people have contributed to the formation of Part I of this book including members of COPP and psychiatric residents at the University of Missouri-Columbia. Thank-you to: Drew Clemens, Jerry Kay, Glen Gabbard, Roy MacKenzie, John Markowitz, Will Sledge, Eva Szigethy, Susan Lazare, Marcia Goin, Michael Hughes, Bob Kimmich, David Goldberg, Jess Wright, Rachel Ritvo, James Griffith, Javad Akhtar, Stephanie Bagby, Alex Jenkins, Myreille Polycarpe, Hope Wagner, Jonathan Colen, Allison Felton, Saleem Kirmani, and Bhaskar Yadurayagowda.

Jennifer Scaia, an excellent graduate research assistant, aided greatly in organizing the text and sharpening its various foci.

The teaching vignettes needed elaboration from experts in several of the subsets of this complex area. With the suggestion of our editor at Norton, Deborah Malmud, three outstanding chapters were developed and incorporated in the book. Michael Thase, also a COPP member, has followed the research literature in combined treatment more carefully than any other writer, having also participated in several complex investigations of combined treatment questions. His chapter presents principles and research conclusions from this vast literature. Michelle Riba with Richard Balon have wondered about, written about, and studied the potentially confusing arrangement variously known as "medical back-up," "pharmacotherapy psychotherapy triangle, " and now most commonly as "split treatment." And Bart Blinder, a long-time member of COPP, undertook the most difficult of the current challenges—trying to make sense of what Freud could not—identifying the apparatus of the brain that supports the functions of the mind.

Psychiatry is the mind-brain profession. Mental health professionals can no longer afford the dichotomy. The authors of this book are firmly committed to healing this conceptual schism in order foster clearer concepts of our patients' problems to lead to better treatment outcomes.

Bernard D. Beitman
Columbia, Missouri
September, 2002

Integrating Psychotherapy and Pharmacotherapy

Introduction

Bernard D. Beitman, M.D.

The mind-brain dichotomy has given way to the beginnings of integration. Treatment of mental illness in the twenty-first century requires "mind-brain" thinking. Psychotherapy influences brain function. Pharmacotherapy influences mind. The time has come in human evolution to recognize and understand the reciprocal relationship between mind and brain, to dissolve the conceptual mind-brain barrier. The increased use of pharmacologic and psychotherapeutic treatments is reflective of the recognition that the brain is the organ of the mind, just as the heart is central to circulation. The disorders treated by psychiatrists and other mental health clinicians are disorders of brain function and often require combined or integrated interventions.

For example, much evidence suggests that pharmacotherapy can influence cognitive functioning in depression (Murphy, Simons, Wetzel, & Lustman, 1984). Pharmacotherapy can control schizophrenic delusions and hallucinations and also increase patients' ability to plan ahead (Tran et al., 1997). Psychotherapy, in its turn, has been shown to affect brain function (see Blinder, Part II).

Both pharmacotherapy and psychotherapy can improve the lives of people with psychiatric disorders (Beitman & Klerman, 1991; Thase, 2000a). The goal now is to maximize the clinical effects of chemical and psychotherapeutic treatments. For some patients, medications provide the opportunity to utilize psychotherapy. For others, medications or psychotherapy alone may be sufficient. Still others may be best served by alternating different treatments. Using both medications and psychotherapy in all patients may not necessarily be most cost-efficient or most effective.

Integrating pharmacotherapy and psychotherapy requires that clinicians attempt to conceptualize the relationship between mind and brain. A patient with posttraumatic stress disorder (PTSD) may have a dysfunctional hippocampus as a result of traumatic events. The brain circuits altered by pharmacotherapy may be separate from those activated by psychotherapy. Or perhaps the two modalities may combine synergistically. In panic disorder involving a possibly hypermetabolic amygdala, psychotherapy may influence prefrontal amygdala circuits, whereas selective serotinin reuptake inhibitors (SSRIs) might "calm" the amygdala through serotonergic activity reaching up from the dorsal raphe nuclei. Medications may help control dysregulated affect, while psychotherapy helps to alter maladaptive interpersonal patterns. Clues are emerging that suggest a neurobiology of transference (Gabbard, 2000; Westen & Gabbard, 2002). Learning can alter the regulation of gene expression through the gene's ability to direct the production of certain proteins (gene transcriptional function) (Kandel, 1998). In the clinic, the potential for relating mind and brain may suddenly appear to those clinicians who are ready to see it. For example:

A 35-year-old single man has been treated with mood stabilizers and antidepressants for mood variability. He wants to discontinue lamotrigine (Lamictal) and begin gabapentin (Neurontin). He is isolated, tends to drink excessively, and intermittently uses cocaine. He refuses to enter psychotherapy despite his ongoing obsessions about his mother, who committed suicide when he was a teenager. He only dimly acknowledges a potential connection between his mother's suicide and his fear of relationships. After beginning the gabapentin he reported odd experiences including seeing visual after-images. He wanted to know if the damage was permanent. His psychiatrist responded, "No, those side effects will go away. But the damage done to your brain by your mother's suicide will not go away unless you do something about it." The patient gradually got the message and sought psychotherapy. As psychotherapy helped him, his concerns about the pharmacological effects diminished.

Useful distinctions can be made among monotherapy, combined therapy, and integrated treatment. During the standard medication-management visit, the psychopharmacologist generally *monitors* symptoms and side effects. During a psychotherapeutically informed pharmacotherapy, the psychopharmacologist *integrates* pharmacotherapy with psychotherapy by addressing directly and indirectly the relationship between them while also inquiring about the patient's personal experiences. Some psychiatrists *combine* pharmacotherapy and psychotherapy by spending a specific time during the session on pharmacotherapy and the remainder on psychotherapy. Others *integrate* psychotherapy with pharmacotherapy by keeping in mind the potential reciprocal relationship between the two treatments—pharmacotherapy can be considered another psychotherapeutic intervention. Under conditions of "split treatment"—pharmacotherapy by one person and psychotherapy by another—the triangle of two clinicians and a patient is generally *combined* rather than *integrated*. This book addresses the myriad of questions that arise from such treatments.

Part I provides an overview of these many issues through active involvement with specific problems and cases. The topics covered include: (1) research in combined treatments, (2) pharmacotherapy during psychotherapy, (3) psychotherapeutic aspects of psychotherapy, (4) the pharmacotherapy-psychotherapy triangle, (5) treatment algorithms for combined treatments, and (6) the neurobiology of psychotherapy.

This part of the book is formatted like *Learning Psychotherapy* (Beitman & Yue, 1999), which includes six modules addressing verbal response modes and intentions, working alliance, inductive reasoning to define patterns, change, resistance, transference and countertransference. Two unpublished modules are available: Module 0, Basic Listening Skills, and Module 7, Termination.* Learning Psychotherapy detailed an integrated model for learning psychotherapy, in which techniques among the major schools of

---

Contact Bernard Beitman at the department of Psychiatry, University of Missouri, Columbia, MO 65201.

psychotherapy are shared. The goals of that program were to teach fundamental skills and concepts that, if well learned, would lead to effective and time-efficient therapy. The foundation of that program, one shared by this book, is the basic ideas, strategies, and techniques common to all the psychotherapies. Integrating pharmacotherapy and psychotherapy requires a basic concept of psychotherapy; it is far too complicated to integrate pharmacotherapy with each of the schools of psychotherapy without first integrating the basics of psychotherapy.

Trainees studying *Learning Psychotherapy* learn to think about the basic skills of psychotherapy. Seminars are analogous to a psychotherapeutic relationship in that the seminar leader, rather than lecturing, facilitates personal growth in psychotherapeutic knowledge and self-understanding through fostering a group-process learning. Instead of passively reading and listening to lectures, trainees are asked to participate in the seminar and to complete homework assignments. This process extends to individual readers as well.

These "Missouri Modules" have been adopted as a basic approach to teaching psychotherapy in more than half the psychiatric training programs in the United States. They have been translated into Spanish and are being used in Canada and Australia. The format is adopted here with the individual reader as well as the seminar leader in mind, and this book may be used on its own or in conjunction with the programs detailed in *Learning Psychotherapy*. Sections are as interactive as possible, with instructions for use both in a formal training setting and for individual readers. In addition, we have included responses from the University of Missouri psychiatric residents, where we have been testing this program. For teachers interested in using Part I as a part of a seminar series, we provide a brief outline of how to plan the series (see Flow Chart for a Ten-Session Seminar Series, p. xxi).

Part II contains detailed elaborations of the key topics of Part I. The first piece, "Conceptual and Empirical Basis for Integrating Psychotherapy and Pharmacotherapy," provides principles and research conclusions to guide clinical practice. Written by Michael Thase, the piece encourages the reader to look beyond easy conclusions like "combined treatment is almost always better" to recognize how difficult it is to draw apparently obvious conclusions. The second piece written by Michelle Riba with Richard Balon, reviews the remarkable complexity (including legal implications) of split treatment. The third piece, "Psychodynamic Neurobiology," written by Barton Blinder, provides many seeds for the growth of our understanding of the relationship between psychotherapy and the brain. Debra Safer contributed excellent editorial details and several useful cases.

The goals of this book are to help readers: (1) become familiar with the findings and limitations of the research literature on combined treatments, (2) learn how to use pharmacotherapy during psychotherapy, (3) learn how to use psychotherapy during pharmacotherapy, (4) learn the issues involved when a patient is treated by both a pharmacotherapist and a psychotherapist, (5) gain an increased understanding of the sequencing of pharmacotherapy and psychotherapy, and (6) begin to conceptualize the neurobiology of psychotherapy. Whether you are an experienced clinician, psychiatric resident, or trainee in the other mental health professions, this book will help you become more conversant with the many issues involved in integrating psychotherapy and pharmacotherapy.

Flow Chart for Ten-Session Seminar Series*		
Training	**Seminar Leader's Tasks**	**Homework Assignments**
Session 1	Go through the book's introduction. Go through introduction to Section 1.	Answer questions to Section 1. Read introduction to Section 2.
Session 2	Discuss answers to questions from Section 1. Review introduction to Section 2.	Vignettes 1–7 of Section 2.
Session 3	Discuss answers to vignettes 1–7 of Section 2.	Vignettes 8–18 of Section 2. Introduction to Section 3.
Session 4	Discuss answers to vignettes 8–18 of Section 2. Review introduction to Section 3.	Vignettes from inpatient and emergency department and outpatient vignettes 1–6 of Section 3.
Session 5	Discuss answers to vignettes from inpatient and emergency department and outpatient vignettes 1–6 of Section 3.	Outpatient vignettes 7–20 of Section 3.
Session 6	Discuss answers to vignettes 7–20 of Section 3.	Vignettes 21–28 of Section 3. Introduction to Section 4.
Session 7	Discuss answers to vignettes 21–28 of Section 3. Review introduction to Section 4.	Vignettes 1–9 of Section 4. Introduction to Section 5.
Session 8	Discuss answers to vignettes 1–9 of Section 4. Review introduction to Section 5.	Vignette of Section 5.
Session 9	Discuss answers to vignette of Section 5.	Read Section 6
Session 10	Discuss Section 6.	X

* For the purposes of clarity, we have formulated this book according to the chronological sequence of the six sections. This flow chart shows the order in which sections should be read and completed within a ten-session seminar series. Because the length of sections varies, some sections require several sessions. At the discretion of the seminar leader, the chapters in Part II should be added to introduction homework readings for Sections 1, 5, and 6.

PART I

Issues, Vignettes, and Commentary

Research in Combined Treatments

INTRODUCTION

The growing research literature in combined treatments has been summarized by Thase (2000a and Part II). Important conclusions from this literature include:

1. Compared to their respective monotherapies, combined treatments do not uniformly produce additive benefits. Because combined treatment is likely to be more costly than monotherapy, before combined treatment is initiated a clear evidence of potential benefit must exist. Practitioners must research and define which subsets of patients are most likely to respond to monotherapy and which are most likely to respond to combined therapy.

    When reviewing the research literature on combined therapy, keep in mind that treatments are split between a psychopharmacologist and a psychotherapist. No attempt is made to *integrate* the treatments, as can be done when one person administers both treatments. Although the data have not yet been gathered, many practitioners believe that integrated treatment is generally superior to split treatment.

2. Some disorders, including schizophrenia, bipolar disorder, and major depression with psychotic features, clearly benefit from pharmacotherapy. Psychotherapy can aid adherence to medication treatment, enhance social and work functioning, and help reduce relapse. In the treatment of schizophrenia, family therapy, social-skills training, and probably cognitive therapy are associated with significant improvement and may offer significant reduction in risk of rehospitalization. For bipolar disorder, a cognitive therapy treatment manual has been developed (Basco & Rush, 1996). Several studies have shown the value of psychosocial treatments for bipolar disorder (Frank et al., 1999; Huxley, Parikh, & Baldessarini, 2000; Miklowitz et al., 2000.)

   Psychosocial interventions sometimes detract from treatment outcomes. For example, a type of individual psychotherapy—the so-called personal therapy—was helpful for schizophrenics who lived with their families. However, this therapy was associated with an increased risk of relapse for patients who lived alone. For men with bipolar disorder, couples therapy was associated with a significant worsening on measures of perceived family support and did not provide benefit on symptomatic measures. Notably, couples therapy was helpful to women with bipolar disorder in these same dimensions (see Thase, 2000a).

3. In controlled clinical trials, the following disorders responded to psychotherapy alone: major (nonbipolar) depressive disorder (e.g., nonpsychotic, nonmelancholic subtype), dysthymia, panic disorder, obsessive-compulsive disorder (OCD), social phobia, generalized anxiety disorder (GAD), bulimia, and primary insomnia. Effective pharmacotherapies also exist for each of these diagnoses. When should treatments be combined? (See Section 6 for treatment algorithms for panic disorder.) The psychotherapies used in these clinical trials have generally been limited to behavioral therapy, cognitive therapy, and interpersonal therapy. Most of these studies primarily measured symptom

reduction without showing clear evidence of continuing effects and improvement in quality of life.

In patients with mild to moderate depression, combined treatment appears to add little to the monotherapies. However, for severely depressed people, the combination is associated with better outcome than either treatment alone. In a large study involving 681 people with chronic depression (Keller et al., 2000), a form of cognitive therapy combined with nefazodone (Serzone) was 25% superior to both monotherapies. Some evidence suggests that patients who respond inadequately to a few months of either monotherapy may find the addition of the other monotherapy quite helpful.

Evidence suggests that marital and family therapy also help treat major depression (Beach, Sandeen, & O'Leary, 1990; Friedman, 1975). Patient vulnerability to depression and family competence to handle the depressive episode are likely to be mutually reinforcing in either positive or negative directions: If the family is able to respond competently, the episode may be shortened; if the family is unable to respond competently, the depressive episode may be prolonged and further impair the family's ability to cope (Keitner & Miller, 1990). Family functioning seems to deteriorate in the 6–12 month period following the diagnosis and treatment of a depressive episode (Keitner et al., 1995). Family intervention may increase the odds of recovery and complement maintenance pharmacotherapy.

Bulimia nervosa appears to best respond to cognitive behavior therapy (CBT) alone or to a combination of CBT and pharmacotherapy. Many different forms of psychotherapy have been used for bulimia nervosa, but studies consistently support behavioral approaches that address the presenting behaviors of binge eating, self-induced vomiting, and laxative abuse. Generally these approaches include detailed food diaries, goal setting, stimulus control (times and conditions under which the patient may eat), response delay (delay between the patient's desire to eat and actually eating), and response prevention (doing something else besides eating) (Beitman, Hall, & Woodward, 1992). A two-stage intervention that begins with psychotherapy and then adds pharmacotherapy also merits study. Another model to consider involves nutritional rehabilitation, psychotherapy, medication, and a support group.

Panic disorder responds well to CBT. Furthermore, CBT combined with antidepressants may be superior by some measures. But evidence suggests that combined treatment using benzodiazepines may be equivalent to psychotherapy alone, perhaps because the patient attributes gains to the benzodiazepine and not to his/her own behavioral efforts.

A significant number of patients with OCD, refuse to accept the behavioral treatment of exposure and response prevention, and perhaps 10–15% refuse serotonergic drugs because of their side effects (Thase, 2000). Patients treated only with SSRIs are much more likely to relapse upon discontinuation of the medication than patients who have completed behavioral treatment alone. Self-help with OCD (Schwartz, 1996), as with other disorders, appears promising in maintaining symptom relief.

4. The research literature will have great difficulty answering the majority of questions regarding which medication is best matched by which psychotherapy. One reason is the tremendous expense of carrying out combined treatment studies. For example, the aforementioned Keller and colleagues depression study, conducted in the United States in the mid-1990s, was estimated to cost $23 million. With at least fifteen different medications and at least three general forms of individual and group psychotherapy—including cognitive, behavioral, interpersonal (Frank, Karp, & Rush, 1993), psychodynamic marital (Friedman, 1975), family and many variations thereof—available for the treatment of depression, the cost to test them clearly

exceeds available resources. And this cost analysis reflects just one diagnostic category!

Table 1.1 lists several research questions awaiting better answers than we now we possess.

5. When compared to psychotherapy, pharmacotherapy has a major disadvantage in that relapse rates after treatment discontinuation are likely to be higher. Cognitive therapy has been used to help patients with panic disorder withdraw from benzodiazepines (Spiegel, Bruce, Gregg, & Nuzzarello, 1994), but no one has systematically attempted to help patients learn from pharmacotherapy by helping them achieve on their own the mind-brain state induced by the external chemical.

TABLE 1.1
Future Research Questions*

- What research approaches should be utilized to permit generalization of integrated/combined treatment findings within a diagnostic category as well as outside a diagnostic category?
- Under what conditions should both medication and psychotherapy be instituted at the outset of treatment?
- Under what conditions should psychotherapy or medications be started first, with the other treatment approach instituted only if the first one fails?
- For which problems and conditions are combined/integrated treatments most cost-effective?
- When is integrated treatment by a psychiatrist superior to split treatment?
- Which psychiatrists are more effective using integrated treatment and why?
- When is split treatment superior to integrated treatment?
- What are the factors critical to the success of split treatment?

After Kay, 2001.

PHARMACOTHERAPY-PSYCHOTHERAPY RESEARCH QUESTIONS

1. List the various ways psychotherapy can positively and negatively affect pharmacotherapy. Also list the ways pharmacotherapy can positively and negatively affect psychotherapy.

    _____

    _____

    _____

    _____

    _____

    _____

2. Design a combined treatment study using five cells. These should include the use of placebo, active drug, and a psychotherapy.

    _____

    _____

    _____

    _____

    _____

    _____

3. List the benefits and limitations of splitting pharmacotherapy between two clinicians instead of having one person conduct both.

    _____

    _____

    _____

    _____

    _____

    _____

ANSWERS/COMMENTARY

1. Psychotherapy positively affects pharmacotherapy by:

    - helping the patient comply with taking medication;

    - building on gains from pharmacotherapy to improve work and social functioning.

    Pharmacotherapy hinders psychotherapy when:

    - the patient becomes satisfied with the drug effects and does not want psychotherapy;

    - the patient and/or the prescriber believe that the patient's taking medication means that the patient cannot be helped by psychotherapy because the problem is too severe;

    - the pill "corrects" the basic problem, making psychotherapy irrelevant (a belief not widely held).

    Pharmacotherapy positively affects psychotherapy by:

    - facilitating the patient's ability to engage in psychotherapy by reducing interfering symptoms;

    - facilitating the patient's ability to self-reflect by reducing the intensity of symptoms distracting the patient from self-reflection;

    - inducing positive expectancies (placebo effect).

    Psychotherapy hinders pharmacotherapy when:

    - too much psychotherapeutic probing diminishes the benefits of the pharmacotherapy (after Klerman, 1991);

    - it leads the patient and/or therapist to ignore the role of biological factors in illness (this could place too much responsibility for change on the patient,

causing him or her to avoid taking potentially helpful and necessary medications).

2. Cell 1: Placebo plus psychotherapy.
   Cell 2. Placebo alone.
   Cell 3. Drug plus psychotherapy.
   Cell 4. Psychotherapy alone.
   Cell 5. Drug alone.

3. Two retrospective studies suggested that the cost of
   having a psychiatrist do both pharmacotherapy and
   psychotherapy was slightly lower than having the treatment split between two clinicians (Goldman et al.,
   1998). A single provider offers a natural integration of
   treatment, less chance of conflicting psychoeducation,
   and no chance of "splitting" between the two clinicians.
   The drawbacks of a single clinician include: lack of the
   psychiatrist's time to use all the current combined treatments and often lack of experience in providing empiri-
   cally tested psychotherapies (assuming those are true
   correlates of positive outcome). Perhaps psychiatrists
   should provide combined treatment for the most complex disorders like comorbid depression with posttraumatic stress disorder or borderline personality disorder.
   Given the vast number of the triangles that exist among
   the psychotherapist, primary care physician, and
   patient, it becomes essential to understand the determinants of such successful relationships. Indifferent or
   poorly executed pharmacotherapy offers little when
   added to well-conducted psychotherapy. It may well be
   that poorly executed psychotherapy adds little to com-
   petent, supportive pharmacotherapy (Thase, 2000a).

RESPONSES OF PSYCHIATRIC RESIDENTS*

A major conceptual problem was discussed: Psychotherapy can
change brain function. Psychiatrists are not psychopharmacolo-

---

* Psychiatric residents' responses throughout the book are from residents at the University
of Missouri, where this program has been tested.

gists *or* psychotherapists. They use both medications and psychotherapy to help patients to change their own brain cognitive-emotion patterns.

Most mental health professionals think in either mind terms (e.g. thoughts, feelings, actions) or in brain terms (e.g. neurochemicals). They have difficulty using mind and brain terms simultaneously. However, the act of taking a pill involves many cognitive, emotional, and behavioral elements. Odd, idiosyncratic responses to the taking of a pill can provide useful ways to understand mental processes. Our trainees had trouble making themselves consider the possibility that reactions to pharmacotherapy could serve as inducing points to maladaptive patterns.

We discussed the psychotherapy of bipolar patients at some length. One trainee asked: "If antidepressants can trigger mania in some depressed bipolar patients, can psychotherapy also do the same thing?" There was general belief that combined treatments are better than monotherapy, but where really was the evidence of that? We reviewed the major criteria for deciding whether or not to use both: diagnosis, severity of symptoms, and patient preference. They wondered how it could be that some patients would come for treatment and not be ready to change.

Trainees struggled with research designs and indications for combined, integrated treatments. They are not used to considering various cells tested against each other. By slowly encouraging them to consider the multiple possibilities they began to grasp the complexity involved with testing combined treatment strategies.

Pharmacotherapy During Psychotherapy

INTRODUCTION

During the process of psychotherapy, pharmacotherapy may be viewed as another psychotherapeutic intervention. Pharmacotherapy includes not only the active drug effect but also the placebo response and the various consequences of offering and prescribing. For example, the offering of medication has a range of meanings for patients, from a gift to a rejection of the interpersonal relationship. The prescription of medications can help to solidify or disrupt the therapeutic bond. Pharmacotherapy can help to clarify maladaptive patterns, initiate change, and maintain change. Medications may influence the duration of therapy, extending or abruptly terminating the course of treatment. Table 2.1 follows a medication perspective through the stages of psychotherapy.

Engagement. Like accurate empathic reflections and effective suggestions, the prescription of medications can help to develop trust and confidence in the therapist. If the medication is effective, confidence and trust are likely to increase. Even if the medication is ineffective, the process of offering the prescription and tracking the medication's effect or lack thereof can provide a medium through which patients and therapists come to know each other

<table>
<tr><td colspan="6" align="center">

TABLE 2.1

Stages of Individual Psychotherapy: A Medication Emphasis*

</td></tr>
</table>

Stage	Engagement	Pattern Search	Change	Termination
Goals	Trust Credibility Self-observer alliance	To define problem patterns that, if changed, would lead to a desirable outcome	1. Relinquish old pattern(s) 2. Initiate new pattern(s) 3. Practice new pattern(s)	To separate efficiently and effectively
Techniques	Effective medications	Homework— idiosyncratic meanings ascribed to medication	Medication-induced change	Continue or discontinue medications
Content	Medication-responsive diagnosis	Does negative response to medication reflect a problem pattern? Times medication taken suggest a problem pattern	Medication effects, or insight around medication use accelerates change	Continue or discontinue medications
Resistance	Are excessive side effects resistant to treatment?	Does pattern of nonadherence to medication regimen reflect a problem pattern?	Do new side effects suggest resistance to change?	Symptom reoccurrence not necessarily indication for medication change

Source: Reprinted from B. D. Beitman (1991), Medications during psychotherapy: Case studies of the reciprocal relationship between psychotherapy process and medication use. In B. D. & G. L. Klerman (Eds.), Integrating pharmacotherapy and psychotherapy. Washington, DC: American Psychiatric Press. See p. 23. Used with permission.

Transference	Physician seen as malevolent or all powerful	Is key interpersonal pattern reflected in meaning of medication?	Unresolved distortions may be signaled by a new medication issue inhibiting change	Desire for new or more medication reflects desire to hold therapist
Countertransference	Physician failure to prescribe appropriately	Medication prescription reflects distorted response to patient	Sudden change in regimen reflects an attempt to undermine change	New medication reflects desire to keep contact

better. However, unexpected major side effects can rupture the relationship. Patients may distrust the meaning of the prescription, and psychiatrists may use medications as a way to punish patients.

Pattern Search. Odd events around the process of offering, prescribing, and ingesting medications can provide "inducing points" for dysfunctional patterns. Refusing to take potentially useful medications, suddenly stopping effective medications, and undiscussed dose escalations or reductions can reveal more generalized malfunctional patterns. For example, perfectionistic patients often expect medications to resolve all their problems, angry patients may attempt to retaliate against their psychiatrist by overdosing on prescribed medications, and frustrated spouses may take pills prescribed to their partner.

Change. The process of pharmacotherapy can be used to help patients to give up old patterns and to initiate and help maintain change. For example, noting the points at which a patient decides to take an "as needed" medication can reveal some critical patterns to be relinquished. An illustration of pharmacotherapy's potential role in initiating change might involve a timid patient's ability to choose a medication against the wishes of others. Pharmacotherapy can also help a person who has started to change but feels anxious or depressed about having done so. Finally, reductions in dose or the discontinuation of medication can help to reinforce positive change by the patient.

Termination. Patients may force termination of therapy around medications. Therapists may force termination and use medications in an attempt to soften the blow. During termination some patients experience a recurrence of symptoms. In these cases, pharmacotherapy may be unnecessary, as symptoms appearing at this time are often short-lived. Issues ostensibly about medications may actually represent a difficulty in separating.

This simplified view of psychotherapy allows pharmacotherapists to push aside the often confusing arguments among the schools of psychotherapy. By recognizing that psychotherapy is based upon a therapeutic relationship that proceeds through stages, psychiatrists can focus on the common factors that influence psychotherapeutic treatment response while also respecting and utilizing useful differences.

In addition, a generic psychotherapeutic view of the processes involved with pharmacotherapy may facilitate a quicker consideration of the possibility that a change in diagnostic symptoms may not necessarily require a shift in pharmacotherapy, but rather a focus on interpersonal/intrapsychic problems.

VIGNETTES

1. The owner of a small family farm, a 30-year-old married man with no children, presented with panic disorder, dysthymia, and social phobia. During the engagement process, he greatly feared his psychiatrist's criticism. Lacking trust in his psychiatrist, he simultaneously was highly self-critical. He wanted his symptoms to go away but he did not want to pay attention to them. He wanted his psychiatrist to make the problems disappear but he did not see that he had any problems except for these various symptoms. He reluctantly took

sertraline (Zoloft) to which, after 8 weeks of treatment, he showed no response in terms of the severity of the target symptoms. Psychotherapy and marital therapy focused on enabling him to assert himself with his wife and to become less fearful of her criticism. He also became less fearful of his psychiatrist. He decided to sell the farm and try a more potentially satisfying job. He also began to feel more deserving of symptom relief and better able to clearly understand how he was contributing to his own problems. He was ready to continue to change. Because he was still moderately depressed, he was offered and accepted paroxetine (Paxil) to which he had a positive response.

Speculate about why he might have responded positively to paroxetine and not to the sertraline, considering movement across the stages of psychotherapeutic change.

_____

_____

_____

_____

_____

_____

2. A 40-year-old very isolated man sought help for self-diagnosed manic-depressive illness. He had a positive family history for manic-depressive illness but he was more paranoid than grandiose. He believed the police were after him and that "blood would run in the streets" with "the coming economic collapse." He insisted that lithium had helped his relatives and he wanted lithium for himself.

What should the psychiatrist do?

_____

_____

_____

_____

_____

_____

3. A 40-year-old man wanted help from a psychiatrist in separating from his agoraphobic and demanding wife. He tended to overindulge her whims. After work done in individual psychotherapy, he began to refuse to respond to each of her many requests. His wife, first angered by this change, requested that he ask his psychiatrist to see her since the psychiatrist was an expert in anxiety disorders. She had made a similar request when he had been in psychotherapy before. The previous psychotherapeutic relationship had been very important to him but he and the previous therapist agreed that the therapist would also see his wife. Subsequently, the therapist felt a conflict of interest in seeing each of them individually and decided to continue only with his wife.

    The current psychiatrist should:

    A. Begin couples therapy.

    B. See her individually.

    C. Look for a maladaptive pattern.

    D. Call her on the phone with him in the office to discuss the request.

4. During the early phase of psychotherapy with a particularly troublesome 28-year-old man, a psychiatrist became frustrated with his patient's demands for medication and continuing reports of shifting side effects that seemed to accompany any medication use. Well-versed in the use of monoamine oxidase inhibitors, she tried the patient on phenelzine (Nardil) and left town

for 2 weeks without clarifying the food restrictions or giving him the name of her backup person.

Explain this usually very responsible psychiatrist's behavior.

_____

_____

_____

_____

_____

_____

5.   After seeing a 23-year-old patient several times, a 28-year-old psychiatric resident found himself the object of her seductive behavior (Langs, 1973). Because the therapist did not believe he could be sexually attractive to women, he could not understand her behavior. He therefore decided to give her antianxiety medication.

How is the patient likely to have responded?

_____

_____

_____

_____

_____

_____

6.   A 35-year-old divorced father of three had several episodes of severe panic and depression after his wife left him for another man. After electro-convulsive therapy (ECT) he remained stable on a variety of anti-depressants. A year after the divorce his 7-year-old daughter was found to have a rare cancer for which the local physicians knew no treatment. He hurriedly

sought other alternatives and, months later found a treatment program that looked promising. However, his sleep became very fitful. His psychiatrist offered him the benzodiazepine flurazepam (Dalmane). Despite the fact that over-the-counter sleeping pills were no longer helpful to him, he refused to accept the flurazepam. He stated that his father was a narcotics agent and to take a controlled substance would be disloyal to him. He then reported that his mother had poisoned his father when the patient was 28 years old.

If benzodiazepines were the only option, how could the psychiatrist convince him that it would be in his best interest to take them temporarily?

_____

_____

_____

_____

_____

_____

7. A 55-year-old woman was referred for psychiatric help for possible depression. She was receiving butalbital (Fiorinal) for intermittent headaches. Her psychiatrist asked her to keep a diary of the times she took the medication. To her surprise she often took it shortly after being criticized or frustrated by a colleague or employer. Interpersonally, she was a great help to others but was absolutely unable to accept nurturance and support for herself. Her inability to accept the psychiatrist's help was becoming increasingly frustrating as well. Near the end of a session, she requested that the psychiatrist rather than the internist give her the butalbital prescription. The psychiatrist reluctantly handed her the script, asking why she was unable to accept emotional understanding and support from anyone. She became furious. In an effort to prove she could

accept personal help, she decided not to fill the prescription; instead, she returned the script the following session and said, "I wanted to prove to you that I could accept your help. I will try to accept your support and concern rather than the pills." She quickly noticed that her mother also was not willing to accept help, although she, too, was a major support to others. She differentiated herself from her mother and began to be more reciprocal in terms of receiving support with others.

The activity around the butalbital script helped the patient:

A. Define a maladaptive pattern and give it up.

B. Give up an old pattern and initiate a new pattern.

C. Initiate a new pattern and maintain it.

D. Maintain a new pattern.

8. A 20-year-old depressed college student was deeply attached to her mother. Any major decisions required a consultation with her mother. Very early in psychotherapy she was offered an antidepressant. She dutifully asked her mother's advice. Her mother replied, "I don't want a drug addict for my daughter!" The patient refused pharmacotherapy. After several more sessions in which her enmeshment with her mother was discussed, she decided to take the antidepressant anyway. She also decided not to tell her mother she had begun this treatment.

What are the possible pharmacological and psychological effects of these decisions?

_____

_____

_____

_____

_____

_____

9. After tolerating her husband's affairs for almost 10 years, a 32-year-old woman decided, with the help of psychotherapy, to divorce him. She resumed her career, became quite successful, and discontinued psychotherapy. After a few months she found herself becoming suicidal. She recognized issues of grief and loss about the marriage. She chose to examine the grief associated with the loss of her marriage in psychotherapy and also to take an antidepressant. She responded positively to the combined treatment.

At what substage of change was the antidepressant offered?

A. Defining a maladaptive pattern.

B. Giving up the old pattern.

C. Initiating the new pattern.

D. Maintaining the new pattern.

10. A psychiatric resident had been seeing an intermittently psychotic 32-year-old man for 18 months. As a therapist and psychopharmacologist, he was deeply invested in this person who had made only modest gains. As the forced termination caused by leaving the residency loomed only a few months away, the patient began to express his anger and sadness at the desertion. The therapist felt increasingly guilty and decided that he should start the patient on a new antiseizure medication that had never been formally tested for psychotic problems.

Identity some of the reasons for the resident to start the patient on this new medication.

_____

_____

_____

_____

_____

_____

11. A 20-year-old college sophomore requested help for her fear about being without a boyfriend, worrying whether her friends liked her, continuing urges to keep her CDs in alphabetical order, and occasional panic attacks. She had no family history of anxiety disorders, depression, or substance abuse. She reported that her father had wanted her to be a basketball player, but she could not make baskets. She felt that she had always disappointed him. After being told about medication treatment for anxiety, she was eager to start begin taking sertraline (Zoloft) and also wanted to know what she could do in addition to medication. She agreed to read *Brain Lock* by Jeffrey Schwartz to learn to deal with her orderliness urges.

After two sessions she reported feeling much less anxious. She was glad to be without a boyfriend and described how she assertively insisted that she and her roommate resolve a recent conflict rather than avoiding it. She had read *Brain Lock* and was better able to step back from her urges by saying to herself: "It's the OCD, not me." She liked the book's idea of a dispassionate observer who could monitor and change her responses to her thoughts and her relationships. She asked how long she would have to stay on the sertraline 75mg.

What would you tell her?

_____

_____

_____

_____

_____

_____

12. Discuss the specific psychotherapeutic issues that many manic patients must face when they are treated successfully with pharmacotherapy.

_____

_____

_____

_____

_____

_____

13. What do you as the therapist do when a patient in psychotherapy responds well to a pill given by a pharmacotherapist and decides to quit psychotherapy?

_____

_____

_____

_____

_____

_____

14. A 32-year-old psychiatrist from Russia, educated in the United States since high school, was leaving her practice for a year-long psychopharmacology fellowship in another city. She discussed termination easily with most of her patients except one—a man who was also from Russia but spoke and understood English relatively poorly. When he struggled with the English words, she volunteered Russian words until she knew he had communicated adequately. She doubted that any other psychiatrist could understand the patient's report of symptoms well enough to make the necessary subtle drug dose changes he seemed to require. The patient had been hospitalized twice for suicide attempts. The psychiatrist was also leaving her two young children in the care of her husband who had been unable to find suitable work despite his Russian law degree. She was concerned that he might find the task of single parenting quite difficult until he and the children joined her several months later. She admitted to herself that "my countertransference is making me avoid bringing up termination."

What countertransference elements were making her avoid termination?

_____

_____

_____

_____

_____

_____

15. Psychiatrists doing integrated treatment should define routine ways of addressing medications during psychotherapy. When, for example, should medications be discussed—at the beginning of the session or at the end?

What are the advantages and disadvantages of each?

_____

_____

_____

_____

_____

_____

16. A 48-year-old, bipolar, married, professional woman with two adult children was reasonably well-maintained on lithium, occasional clonazepam (Klonopin), and divalproex sodium (Depakote). In psychotherapy she struggled with her husband's aloofness and her geographical distance from her aging mother, who was being exploited by her alcoholic son (the patient's brother). For various reasons her mother decided to move to the patient's town, much to the patient's delight. The patient began to fantasize about shared shopping trips, restaurant meals, and movies. But then her mother changed her mind. Subsequently, the patient had difficulty sleeping, appeared agitated at work, and could not concentrate. During her next session she demanded medication to "stop me from feeling so bad."

    What would you do?

    _____

    _____

    _____

    _____

    _____

17. A 20-year-old college student presented with major depression, OCD, panic disorder, and obsessive-compulsive personality traits (after Mintz, in press). His obsessive ruminations were unbearable to his family, who tried to "hush" him. But he could not stop his obsessive thinking despite multiple trials of antidepressants, mood stabilizers, antipsychotics, and anxiolytics. When his psychiatrist (who was also his therapist) started him on an antidepressant and mood stabilizer he began to complain of fatigue and intolerable emotional deadness. During therapy, whenever

he felt slighted by the therapist, he would make statements like: "Oh, just put me in a cage and throw a blanket over me," or "Just take the top of my head and scoop my brains out," or "Can't you just turn me into a zombie?" He stopped the medication.

Why did he stop the medication?

_____

_____

_____

_____

_____

_____

18. A late-adolescent boy refused to manage his own medications, instead relying upon his parents to provide them both morning and evening. He was angry with his parents for what he perceived as their neglect of him. On a previous occasion he had stopped his medications and had to be hospitalized because of a furious mania.

What could be the meaning of having his parents provide him with medications, and what should be the focus of therapy?

_____

_____

_____

_____

_____

_____

SUGGESTED ANSWERS/COMMENTARY

1.   After not being sure what to do when given the sertraline, the patient was ready to change when given the paroxetine. Refer to Table 2.1, to see that at first the patient had not engaged with the psychiatrist and was not sure what to change. When he was offered paroxetine, he had moved through the stages of the psychotherapy relationship and seemed ready to use it to change.

2.   The psychiatrist gave him lithium. During the subsequent 18 months the patient delivered diatribes against the government and against the local police department. In between these monologues, they were able to discuss lithium side effects and blood levels although there was no apparent change in his delusions or mood. Through these monologues they were, however, able to explore his paranoid delusions. Finally he accepted risperidone. As sometimes happens when a person relinquishes long-held beliefs, he became depressed when he gave up his delusions. After recovery he began to embark on relationships with others.

3.   C. The psychiatrist emphatically refused to see the wife and pointed out previous examples of the patient's compliance with her demands. "Maybe you could speak with her on the phone," the patient insisted. After several more runs at this pattern, the patient accepted that the therapist was modeling behavior he needed to copy. He finally did learn to say "No!" to his wife. They divorced. Her agoraphobia lessened after the divorce.

4.   The patient called to inquire about side effects and found no one to answer his questions. The therapist's behavior appeared to be the product of unconscious anger at the difficult patient. The patient quit therapy soon after. The psychiatrist declined to examine her motivations in this case.

5.   The patient became confused, began to doubt the therapist's ability to help her, and left therapy.

6. The psychiatrist said: "I asked him if I might speak to his father in him. He agreed. I told 'his father' that his son needed these medications temporarily, perhaps in part for the terrible impact his wife's actions had on his son. 'He needs to sleep. He is exhausted and frightened.' The patient stated that his father would accept these reasons. He took the medication for a few weeks with less guilt and slept better."

7. B.

8. She benefitted not only from the pharmacological action of the antidepressant but also from the boundary she established between her mother and herself. This reciprocal effect spiraled into a clear separation from her mother and a consequent establishment of a firm sense of self. After 18 months she discontinued the antidepressant and maintained most of her gains for the subsequent 6 months of follow-up.

9. D. To maintain ability to function well outside the marriage. Or A if unresolved grief from the loss of the marriage is determined to be interfering with her ability to function independently.

10. Medications appeared to be the only way to continue contact in a symbolic way after they separated physically, although these new medications offered a low possibility of "cure." The gesture also helped to relieve the resident's guilt about leaving and offered a way to avoid having to confront directly the pain that termination was causing both of them.

11. With no family history and a very rapid response to the SSRI, she would probably need to be on medication for at most 6–9 months. Because she used her own strong psychological abilities to retrain her brain to respond differently to relationship problems and OCD urges, she is likely to maintain these changes without medication. She could always begin taking it again if, under stress, she fell back into old patterns of thinking.

12. Bipolar patients are likely to have several psychotherapeutic issues, including:

Loss of the pleasure of mania. Manic patients often consider their mania pleasurable, a kind of endogenous amphetamine. During these times they have been creative, funny, full of energy, and the center of much attention. The loss of these pleasurable states of mind can be very painful.

Fear of mood changes. Because their depressive episodes can be so difficult and mania problematic, too, many bipolar patients become excessively frightened by mood changes, fearing that a full-blown depressive or manic episode might be coming on. Even normal sadness and grief reactions can engender episodes of intense anxiety that may help to bring on the feared consequence.

Alienation of friends and family. Manic and depressive episodes can alienate friends and family, disrupting long-held, important social connections. Psychotherapy may need to be directed at mourning these illness-induced losses.

Missing developmental tasks. Bipolar adolescents may miss confronting and mastering developmental tasks because they, like drug abusers, have been removed from the normal flow of change.

Denial of illness. Because of these and other difficulties associated with having bipolar affective disorder, these people often deny that they have a problem. Some may remember only the pleasure and not the problems associated with being manic.

13. Even though a psychotherapist might be convinced that psychotherapy is the better treatment, if the patient is not interested in using this means of change, there can be no argument for psychotherapy. Let the patient decide!

14. The fears that her Russian patient might not make it without her were exaggerated by her fears that her Russian husband also might not make it without her.

15. Opening the session with medication monitoring may bias the content in an unproductive way. On the other hand, it may bring up critical issues regarding not only side effects and symptoms but also various distortions

and problems around taking medications. Leaving medications issues to the end may cause key problems to be overlooked or shorten discussion about them. Some clinicians decide to wait to see if and when medication issues should be addressed during the course of the session.

16. Address the grief of the loss of her mother's companionship and the anger she felt that her brother would keep exploiting her mother. When the patient recognized that her symptoms were triggered by a kind of grief, she began to mourn the loss with minimal use of clonazepam.

17. The patient believed that the psychiatrist was prescribing medication in order to silence him as his family members had tried to do: He agreed to take the medication in the context of psychotherapy focusing on his ability to trust and gain support from people.

18. The angry, rebellious young man could be expressing his resentment toward authority by refusing to manage his own medications while simultaneously eliciting support and concern from his parents. An increasing willingness to manage his own medications would hopefully reflect an increasing independence from his parent and an ability to depend upon them in a more mature way. Therapy should focus on helping him become more responsible for his own treatment.

RESPONSES OF PSYCHIATRIC RESIDENTS

Vignette #2 generated much discussion. A few could see the value of using lithium for engagement while several others felt uncomfortable without a secure diagnosis. When is it wise to engage and a patient to use a medication that is unlikely to relieve symptomology? Several clearly stated they would not use a benzodiazepine in this way.

Vignette #3 reminded one trainee of a case of hers. How does one manage each individual relationship and the couple as well?

Vignette #4 frightened a few residents because of the medical legal implications of not providing information and backup. Could countertransference be that strong? Was the psychiatrist having trouble with demanding men in her own life?

Vignette #5 raised the issue of resident need for psychotherapy. Should such a service be started and continued by residents, and should there be lower fees for residents in psychotherapy?

Regarding vignette #6, trainees discussed the concept of using good intentions of the deceased person to help patients in the future.

The discussion of vignette #7 addressed giving up an old pattern and initiating a new pattern. Trainees suggested that one may not give up an old pattern without initiating a new one in its place. For instance, an ex-smoker may initiate a new pattern to carry out during the time that previously was reserved for smoking.

Regarding vignette #8, trainees struggled to grasp the idea that reactions to the process of pharmacotherapy could serve as inducing points for psychological patterns. Residents speculated that even if the patient did not tell her mother about accepting pharmacotherapy, her behavior with her mother would still be changed and could lead to further changes. They discussed generally how changes in one part of a system can cause other changes in the system.

Trainees felt that vignette #9 had two possible answers: A and B. Becoming suicidal and returning to the therapist helped to define the maladaptive pattern of maintaining relationships that had been part of her marriage. They speculated that pharmacotherapy might have been used to avoid discussing the psychological issues of grief and loss associated with the termination of therapy.

Vignette #10 provoked trainees to consider how the offer of a pill could not only be an attempt by the psychiatric resident to reduce his guilt about not helping his patient sufficiently but also be a way to avoid the painful discussion of termination.

Vignette #11 stirred debate about when and how to stop effective medications. Vignette #12 reminded them that manic patients suffer the consequences of their mood swings. Adolescents with bipolar disorder elicited heated discussion. Like diabetic adolescents, they fight parental influence and stop their medications. Vignette #13 stimulated our psychopharmacology-reigns-supreme resident to gloat over the power of pills versus the power of talk. "Drug reps like you," commented another. Vignette #14 struck home for residents from other countries. They recognized their own desire to favor people from their homes over locally born patients. Vignette #16 again forced them to think about psychosocial influences on mood states: "How can we be sensitive to these issues in brief medication visits?" Vignette #17 required that they think of themselves as transference objects whether they like it or not. Several did not like it. "Too much thinking," they said.

Psychotherapy During Pharmacotherapy

INTRODUCTION

Many psychiatric encounters involve the prescription and discussion of medication. Such appointments usually last anywhere from 10 to 30 minutes. Often, the discussion of side effects and symptoms takes little more than 5 of these minutes. The remainder of the time can be used for a number of purposes. The primary purpose of most medication visits is to encourage the patient to continue to adhere to the prescribed medication regimen. Several lines of evidence suggest that "the drug delivery system"(e.g., the doctor/patient relationship) is a crucial variable in outcomes; the better the relationship the higher likelihood of a positive response to medication (Krupnick et al., 1996). Without a relationship that focuses on more than solely monitoring symptoms and side effects, outcome is poor (Murphy, Carney, Knesevich, Wetzel, & Whitworth, 1995).

The therapeutic alliance may help to create a "holding" environment in which the acceptance of taking a drug can be enhanced. Within the context of a supportive and collaborative relationship concerns—such as fear of dependence on medication, resistance, demoralization regarding the delayed or variable effects of medication, and difficulty tolerating the discomforts of side effects—can be addressed and worked through (Krupnick et al., 1996).

Further evidence of the importance of the relationship comes from a study of end-of-residency transfer of care for psychopharmacology patients. Departing residents reported that after notification of transfer, about 20% of their patients worsened, 32% required medication changes, and about 10% decided to quit their medications. Residents receiving these patients reported that 10% worsened, 7% required medication changes, and more than 10% decided to stop their medication (Mischoulon, Rosenbaum, & Messner, 2000).

Finally, malpractice claims involving medication errors rose sharply in the late 1990s; patients were angry about the way their doctors hurried them out of the room to maximize revenue (Zwillig, 1999). "Medication management," unlike the psychotherapy codes that include psychotherapy and medication management (i.e., the Evaluation and Management codes), has no minimum time requirement.

Pharmacotherapists often use the term "supportive psychotherapy" to describe the nonmedication aspects of their interactions. In addition to encouraging adherence to medication regimens, time may be spent solidifying the relationship by asking about current life events and stressors as well as encouraging adaptive responses that have been made more possible by positive medication responses. Supportive psychotherapy does not usually target change of maladaptive patterns but rather focuses on marshaling current resources to maintain current gains.

The manner in which patients respond to the process of pharmacotherapy can illustrate maladaptive interpersonal and intrapsychic problems. For example, the perfectionistic patient may expect the medication to act "perfectly" and, as happens in other aspects of his or her life, be disappointed by its effectiveness. These patterns may be illustrated at any point during the process—from the initial suggestion of a pill to problems in continuing taking the pills. However, the primary purpose of the pharmacotherapy relationship is not to discover psychological patterns but instead to initiate and maintain effective pharmacotherapy. Defining problematic patterns may, however, help patients to continue taking medications.

Ideally, the pharmacotherapist suggests a treatment course, the patient accepts and takes the medications as prescribed, the patient then feels better, and finally the two decide how long the patient should remain on medications. In reality the process is not that simple. For instance:

1. Some patients are afraid to take pills, fearing side effects, addiction, or the negative meaning of taking psychiatric drugs.
2. Some are excessively sensitive to side effects either because they overinterpret minor physical sensations or because they truly are highly reactive physiologically to many different ingested chemicals.
3. Some stop taking their pills when their symptoms improve because they assume they will simply continue to feel better. Some refuse to stop because they are afraid they will feel worse again.

Psychotherapeutic principles can be useful in helping people begin medications, handle side effects, and maintain treatment (Ward, 1991). Kemp, Kirov, Everitt, Hayard, and David (1998) developed "compliance therapy," a systematic approach to the psychotherapeutic aspects of pharmacotherapy. Their approach is summarized in Table 3.1.

A cognitive approach focuses directly on the specific thoughts that interfere with taking medications. By assuming that compliance will likely be a problem for patients, psychopharmacologists can assess the likelihood of noncompliance by directly asking patients (after Beck, 2001):

- How likely are you to take this medication every day, in the way it is prescribed at breakfast and bedtime (or as otherwise prescribed)?
- How likely is it that the medication will help you?
- What might get in the way of your taking it (for example, cost, actually going to the pharmacy, remembering to take it)?
- Will your family/friends/roommates support your taking it?
- How will you remember to take it?

TABLE 3.1
Compliance Therapy

Phase I: Initiation of treatment

1. Review patient's illness history to summarize patient's conceptualization of the illness and expectations of psychopharmacology (help shape the patient's expectations to be realistic—some expect miracles, others expect little—and offer reasonable time frames for response).

2. Predict possible side effects (depending on suggestibility of patient and likelihood that patient will seek excessive information) and withdrawal symptoms.

3. Acknowledge negative treatment experiences (e.g., lack of understanding or support of previous psychopharmacologist; if there were problems, predict possibility of recurrence in current relationship and the hope that they might be discussed before patient terminates).

4. Address patient's denial of illness or need for treatment with inquiry into negative social consequences or lifestyle disruptions (e.g., ask why others might think there is a problem).

5. Compare mental illness and psychopharmacology to other medical problems and drugs like diabetes and insulin. For example, describe the need to increase serotonin activity in the raphe nuclei to reduce amygdala firing.

Phase II: Early treatment

1. Look for, predict, and discuss common misperceptions about treatment, including:
   A. Meaning of medications ("Taking medications means I am weak" or "I should be able to do this on my own").
   B. Fear of addiction to medication.
   C. Loss of control over behavior (paranoid people fear becoming less vigilant).
   D. Loss of personality (numbing of emotional responses to others, loss of manic creativity).
   E. Confusion of symptoms and side effects (e.g., some anxiety patients treated with antidepressants experience an increase in anxiety symptoms during the first weeks).

2. Discuss and clarify the following topics:

    A.   Natural tendency to stop medication when symptoms improve (in spite of the fact that adequate treatment requires longer periods of medication).

    B.   Identity as a "sick person."

    C.   Benefits and drawbacks of treatment (e.g., increased sleepiness, but also less tension and agitation). Some patients become so focused on potential side effects that they will take no medications. Sexual side effects are a major concern for many people. The threat of weight gain prohibits many women from trying many medications.

3.   Focus on both direct and indirect benefits of treatment (medication may not improve all symptoms, but can improve social interactions).

4.   Develop various ways to enhance compliance:

    A.   Examine practical behavioral changes to ensure compliance (e.g., using a pill counter, switching the dose to twice a day instead of three times a day, making pill taking part of other daily routines).

    B.   Use metaphors that suggest positive associations with medication such as "a protective layer," or "an insurance policy," or "a vaccine" (as against the flu). One anxious patient described effective gabapentin as a "brain coat."

    C.   Portray poor compliance as negatively affecting patient in terms of needs, lifestyles, and goals (e.g., without medication, patient is much more disorganized and unreliable at work).

5.   Attempt to link medication cessation with relapse.

Phase III: Maintenance

1.   Use normalizing rationales to combat stigma (e.g., reframing use of medication as a freely chosen strategy to enhance the quality of life).

2.   Portray mental illness as analogous to some physical illnesses by underscoring that physical illnesses require maintenance treatment (e.g., diabetics require insulin, people with hypertension sometimes require multiple medications).

3.   Highlight prevalence of illness with examples of famous sufferers (e.g., Abraham Lincoln was bipolar; see Jamison, 1993).

4.   Reframe the use of medication as:

    A.   A freely chosen strategy.

B. A treatment that enhances the quality of life.
C. A personal decision.
D. Objectively effective: use checklists for symptoms (e.g., anxiety and/or depression) to demonstrate changes from beginning treatment.
5. Focus on importance of staying well:
A. To reach self-identified goals.
B. To maintain valued sources of fulfillment.
6. Discuss possibilities of stopping medication (when episode of depression is over, when psychological triggers for anxiety are well handled, or when life stressors are minimized).
7. Identify characteristics of prodromal symptoms (e.g., decreased sleeping preceding a manic episode, decreased ability to remember).
8. Emphasize early intervention to prevent more serious episodes.
9. Learn to differentiate normal emotional responses from indicators for symptomatic worsening.

To explore the problems with compliance even further, Beck (2001) recommended helping patients visualize the sequence by which medications are to be taken. Obstacles to adherence are identified as well, followed by problem-solving and/or replacing dysfunctional thinking with more adaptive forms. She offers the following case example:

Mr. P, a 23-year-old college student, knew he should take a mood stabilizer and an antidepressant to help him with his mood swings. However, he expressed some ambivalence to his psychiatrist:

Dr. B: (summarizing) So you will get the medicine from the drug store on the way home today, but you think you might not actually end up taking it?
Mr. P: Yeah.
Dr. B: Can you imagine now that it's bedtime and you remember you're supposed to be taking the first dose?
Mr. P: (nods)
Dr. B: Where are you?

Mr. P: In the bathroom. Brushing my teeth.

Dr. B: And how are you feeling?

Mr. P: Tired, worried.

Dr. B: And what is going through your mind?

Mr. P: What if it has a bad effect on me? It could make me zombie out.

Dr. B: Anything else?

Mr. P: Yeah. What if Jim [one of Mr. P's housemates] finds out I'm taking it? He might go around telling everyone.

Together they then addressed the practical problem of where to keep the pills and role-played what to say to himself about "being zombied out" ("the likelihood of that happening is very small with this dose of this medication") and what to say if his housemate saw him taking medications ("they are helping me keep my mind on the schoolwork I need to do") (Beck, 2001, pp. 123–124).

In addition, simple behavioral suggestions can enhance compliance. Many patients have trouble remembering a midday dosage while being regular with morning and night dosages. Wristwatch alarms, medication logs, and pill dispensers can help. If they don't, a change to a medication given twice daily should be considered. However, some compliance problems are deeply rooted in longstanding beliefs that become applied to the pharmacotherapy situation. Patients who seek perfect answers to their problems, are unable to trust the psychopharmacologist's advice, or have pervasive beliefs that they do not deserve to feel better will require more psychotherapeutic effort to overcome noncompliance.

VIGNETTES

Inpatient Case

1. A 26-year-old married woman with a history of bipolar affective disorder is admitted to the inpatient unit for depression with suicidal ideation. While you are introducing yourself, her husband, who is present in the room, asks you about placing the patient on

oxcarbazepine (Trileptal) because he's heard it is less dangerous during pregnancy. You notice that the patient looks down while he is talking. You agree that the patient's medications probably need adjustment and think consideration of oxcarbazepine sounds reasonable.

What psychological aspects of the decision should be considered? Of note, the patient is not currently pregnant.

_____

_____

_____

_____

_____

Emergency Department Cases

1. A 43-year-old married a woman with no prior psychiatric history arrives in the emergency department complaining of acute-onset chest pain that awakened her from sleep. Her medical workup is negative and her symptoms improve with lorazepam (Ativan). You are asked to evaluate for panic disorder.

    While taking the history, you find that the patient recently returned to work now that her children are school age. However, the patient had to discontinue working shortly after commencing work due to anxiety symptoms.

    The patient refuses your referral to the psychiatric outpatient clinic for follow-up, stating that her symptoms are purely physical and that the doctors must have missed something.

    What psychological considerations might you have?

_____

_____

_____

_____

_____

_____

2.   A 27-year-old married man, a graduate student in busi-
      ness school, is admitted to the hospital for a manic
      episode. He was walking naked in the streets talking
      loudly about "Jesus Christ." The patient refuses medica-
      tions, stating that nothing is wrong with him. He tells
      you repeatedly that he is the smartest MBA student in
      his school. The following day, he approaches you to ask
      about a research study that one of the other patients on
      the unit had mentioned. The study is intended for
      patients with bipolar disorder and you believe the
      patient might benefit from participating.

      What might you say to him?

      _____

      _____

      _____

      _____

      _____

      _____

3.   An 18-year-old woman is admitted to the inpatient
      ward with anorexia nervosa and depression. The
      patient is not gaining much weight and appears
      increasingly depressed. You and your team feel a trial of
      an antidepressant is warranted, but the patient refuses,
      saying she doesn't want medication and "doesn't care
      anyway" about feeling happier.

Through your work with this patient you notice that one of the few things she seems to have enjoyed prior to admission was her job working as an assistant in a daycare center. She visibly brightens when talking about her love of babies.

How might this history help you in explaining the risks/benefits of medications to this patient?

_____

_____

_____

_____

_____

_____

Outpatient Cases

1.　A 37-year-old man with panic disorder and agoraphobia received effective treatment of his symptoms with imipramine (Tofranil). His wife often complained that part of their marital difficulty was due to his overlooking obvious problems in their marriage. Three months after his treatment, on a business trip to Hawaii, he felt so good that he decided to stop the medication. Six days later on his return home he had a major panic attack on the plane. He attributed the attack to his dislike of having to return home.

There probably was another reason—one that could illustrate an interesting pattern of his. What might it be?

_____

_____

_____

_____

_____

_____

2. A 21-year-old woman with panic disorder and agora-
    phobia preferred to use phenelzine over imipramine
    because she did not want to have a dry mouth, be
    sedated, or possibly have orthostatic hypotension. She
    also refused to consider SSRIs (selective serotonin
    reuptake inhibitors) due to fear of sexual side effects.
    She was willing to follow the monoamine oxidase
    inhibitor dietary restrictions and work with her psychi-
    atrist in psychotherapy. She responded very positively
    with a reduction in panic and phobic avoidance.
    Unfortunately, however, she became phobic not only of
    foods containing cheese but also of many other foods.
    She stopped the phenelzine but still would not eat a
    wide variety of foods because of her new set of phobias.
    She refused to follow her psychiatrist's suggestion to
    utilize birth control and became pregnant. She quit
    psychotherapy.

    Speculate about what led to this patient-initiated ter-
    mination.

    _____

    _____

    _____

    _____

    _____

    _____

3. A 43-year-old mother of three children, married since
    age 17, was seen by neurologist for a stroke caused by
    an intracranial bleed. She made a remarkable recovery
    but was referred to a psychiatrist for treatment of her
    agoraphobia and severe depression. She benefitted

greatly from a combination of antidepressants, benzodiazepines, and psychotherapy. She and the psychiatrist not only examined the patient's "what if . . ." fears but also her lack of assertiveness with her husband, her tendency to give to others without asking for anything in return, and the consequent lack of concern shown her by her now-grown children.

After 3 years she remained on medications because she had a history of recurrent depression. She was seen in follow-up visits about every 3 months. During one of these meetings she reported yet another problem that appeared beyond her control. Somewhat irritated, her psychiatrist said, "It seems like something negative repeatedly happens and because of that we will need to keep meeting." To her, this remark sounded very much like her husband's complaints that most problems were her fault. She became angry but did not report her reaction during the session. Instead she talked about how hard it would be if she had to see another therapist. She wondered if the psychiatrist liked her and felt that he did not. She was upset that he might leave the area sometime in the future. The next day she called to say she was stopping her medications.

Why was she thinking about stopping the medications?

_____

_____

_____

_____

_____

_____

4. A 24-year-old college senior was depressed and anxious. She loved her fiancé but was not sure she could enjoy their relationship. She was having difficulty concentrating at school, her grades were falling, and she was "faking" being happy. Just like her mother, she

could convince people she was fine when actually she was miserable inside. Her mother had a history of major depression and had responded very positively to paroxetine 10mg. Her maternal grandfather had committed suicide and a cousin had severe OCD (obsessive–compulsive disorder). She thought a maternal aunt had been hospitalized for depression. In retrospect, she felt she had been depressed more often than not since she was about 13.

The patient started on paroxetine and had a dramatic positive response. She felt normal. She wanted to know about future treatment. Should she stay on the medication and begin psychotherapy? How long should she be on the medication?

What would you tell her?

_____

_____

_____

_____

_____

_____

5. A 53-year-old mother of three children wanted help with depression and intense anxiety. At the time of the initial evaluation, she was in the midst of struggling to gain custody of her two grandchildren, who were being taken away from her daughter because of the daughter's inability to care for them. She had tried to make her daughter's life with them better by having all three of them move in with her, but could not. She was treated with sertraline 50mg and clonazepam 0.5mg b.i.d.

During her medication visits, she grieved the loss of the grandchildren, who were sent to live with other relatives out of town. She rebuked herself for failing to keep them with her. However, she was able to return to work and began socializing again. No longer was she staying home, going from "bed to couch," eating poorly, and feeling extremely unmotivated. She discontinued follow-up after a year and seven medication appointments.

She returned 3 years later due to a recurrence of her depressive symptoms. She had been off all medications for 2 years. Her younger son's moving back in with her triggered the depressive reaction. He would not follow probation restrictions and was sent to a halfway house and then to jail again. She was very frustrated with his inability to care for himself. She could not make his life better.

Further review of her history revealed that 9 years earlier her older son had died of AIDS. She had done all she could to keep him alive. As he was dying, she experienced her first major depressive episode. She could not save him.

She began again on sertraline and clonazepam and gradually recovered sufficient function to return to work.

What pattern seemed to trigger her depressive episodes?

_____

_____

_____

_____

_____

_____

6.   A 40-year-old accountant for a Midwest company comes in for treatment for depression. He has been married for 20 years and has three children. His 16-year-old is being treated for ADHD (attention deficit hyperactivity disorder); his 14-year-old has spina bifida and behavioral problems. His 12-year-old is

doing very well in school and appears not to be a problem for his family. The patient is being treated by the same psychiatrist for 2 years. His sessions last 20 minutes, with seven sessions per year. Visits focus on pharmacotherapy for the patient's recurrent depression. The patient is generally maintained on paroxetine 30mg, with 60mg required during particularly difficult periods.

The patient came late to a session for about the fourth time. The psychiatrist asked him what was going on. He stated that he was caught up with the needs of some of his clients with whom he was consulting in another town, and rather than cut off the interview, he decided to stay as long as they needed him. He had many complaints about the difficulties with his wife but had continued to try to accommodate her wishes.

What pattern is being illustrated during these medication checks?

_____

_____

_____

_____

_____

_____

7. A 29-year-old man came to pharmacotherapy evaluation for social anxiety. He feared not living up to the expectations of others. He had previously taken paroxetine for this problem but because of significant sexual side effects, he discontinued it. However, the evaluating psychiatrist did not elicit this history. The psychiatrist had samples of paroxetine readily available and enthusiastically recommended it for the patient. The patient took the samples but did not take the pills.

Why did he accept the pills when he intended not to take them?

_____

_____

_____

_____

_____

_____

8.   A 34-year-old cocaine addict released from prison presented with major depression. She responded very well to sertraline 50mg. She stated: "I felt much better. No depression, more energy, more optimistic. But I stopped it because I was no longer interested in sex and could not have an orgasm."

Speculate about this decision.

_____

_____

_____

_____

_____

_____

9.   A 48-year-old Vietnam War veteran had become a mercenary in Africa after the war. Subsequently, he hired himself out to governments in other parts of the world to help the armies to keep the civilian populations from rebelling. He stated that he had tried many medications for his depressive symptoms and none had worked. He doubted that anything could help him. His psychopharmacologist empathetically concurred with him that nothing was likely to help.

Speculate about the reasons for this belief.

_____

_____

_____

_____

_____

_____

10. A 35-year-old alcoholic with polysubstance abuse had OCD symptoms but refused to take an SSRI for this problem and did not want to go through the rigors of behavioral therapy. He was afraid of the pills, and the behavior therapy (exposure and response prevention) seemed too difficult.

Give several possible reasons for his reluctance to take medications.

_____

_____

_____

_____

_____

_____

11. A 35-year-old nurse is terrified of taking any medications for his severe panic disorder and agoraphobia. He tried a low dose of imipramine and felt dizzy. Yet he was having several panic attacks per day, at least one of which is typically very severe. He could not work and could not travel. His psychopharmacologist began with a very low dose of gabapentin and asked him to increase the dose very slowly. When the patient asked about side effects, the physician told him that

"Gabapentin is associated with growing hairs on the palms of the hands." The patient laughed.

What two psychotherapeutic principles were being used in the psychopharmacologist's treatment?

_____

_____

_____

_____

_____

_____

12. A 45-year-old depressed man had spent the past 4 years seeing a variety of psychiatrists and primary-care physicians, each of whom had given him antidepressants, each of which he had stopped. When he started seeing a new psychiatrist, he again asked for antidepressants.

What is the pattern and what therapeutic approaches might be considered?

_____

_____

_____

_____

_____

_____

13. A 48-year-old man had been depressed for more than 6 months. He had sought treatment from his primary-care physician, who had prescribed trazodone (Desyrel) for sleep and venlafaxine (Effexor) for depression. He had difficulty gaining erections and

had tried paroxetine with no success. He refused to try other SSRIs because of the sexual side effects. His sleep did not improve, nor did his depressive symptoms. He sought psychiatric help and was placed on mirtazapine (Remeron) 15mg. He slept better though he was groggy during the day. During the next session, his psychiatrist—without reviewing the chart—discussed other possible medications. He suggested both venlafaxine and trazodone. The patient looked disappointed. They then decided simply to raise the mirtazapine because at higher doses it can be less sedating.

The psychiatrist felt guilty about not having remembered the patient's previous medications.

What would you do in this situation?

_____

_____

_____

_____

_____

_____

14.   A 28-year-old psychiatric resident was anxious in his dealings with his supervisors and colleagues. He seemed uncertain of his abilities to help patients. Very few of his patients were successfully treated with pharmacotherapy.

Speculate about the reasons.

_____

_____

_____

_____

_____

_____

15. What are some of the possible reasons patients would become so focused on potential side effects that they refused to take medications?

_____

_____

_____

_____

_____

_____

16. A 68-year-old man became very depressed after the death of his wife. He returned to the place to which they had vacationed each summer for the past 20 years. "Why go there anymore?" he said to himself. "She's not here to enjoy it with me." At the urging of his children he sought psychiatric help. Sertraline and trazodone were remarkably helpful to him. After a few months he decided to stop.

What are some of the possible reasons he discontinued his medications?

_____

_____

_____

_____

_____

_____

17. You are leaving your clinic and must terminate with approximately sixteen patients with whom you have been doing psychopharmacotherapy. What can you do

to smooth their transition to another psychopharmacologist?

_____

_____

_____

_____

_____

_____

18. During pharmacotherapy patients often bring up problems in their lives. For the following questions there are
no "right" answers. The questions are intended to
prompt you to clarify how you would handle the situations. What would you do if a patient you are treating
with medications said (adapted from Sabo & Rand,
2000)

"I know we have been trying to find the right combination of medications to help me to cope with my depression, but I've been thinking about a bus trip our high
school class took and it's bothering me."

_____

_____

_____

_____

_____

_____

"The medications you have prescribed for me have
helped a great deal but I'm also thinking that if my husband doesn't stop criticizing me and doesn't start
spending more quality time with me and the kids, I will
get depressed again."

_____

_____

_____

_____

_____

_____

"My parents want to know more about what is going on with your treatment of me."

_____

_____

_____

_____

_____

_____

19.   A lawyer's boss insisted that he seek help for reducing his quick, scathing comments that were making him lose credibility in the downsizing firm (adapted from Sabo & Rand, 2000). For the past few months he had been overeating and sleeping poorly. He also lost interest in sex and felt overwhelmed when trying to solve the simplest problems. He had two small children, and his wife had recently been diagnosed with a serious, potentially debilitating disease. He wanted one of the new antidepressants. During the interview the psychiatrist noted that the patient listened well and was able to consider other perspectives. He could shift mood states with his shifts in perspective. The psychiatrist explained his depressive symptoms as due to stressors at work and with his wife. The psychiatrist suggested that the patient check out his status with others in the firm whom he could trust. After writing a script for an SSRI and going over the potential side effects, he mentioned that psychotherapy could also be helpful for depressed people. Predict what happened in this case (the real outcome is likely to surprise you).

_____

_____

_____

_____

_____

20. A psychiatrist told his pharmacotherapy patient that he was leaving the clinic in 2 months. The patient replied, "I will miss you. I wish I could go to Kansas City with you." The psychiatrist said, "The next person is just as good as I am."

Describe the potential countertransference reasons for this response and the patient's probable emotional reactions.

_____

_____

_____

_____

_____

21. A 38-year-old woman is referred to you by her previous psychiatrist, who had moved to another city. The patient has a long mental health treatment career. She has fired many psychiatrists and psychotherapists, has been psychiatrically hospitalized more than 20 times for suicidal ideation and attempts, and has tried many different medications with very limited success. She describes herself as having many depressive episodes and being borderline ("But I've had plenty of therapy and am much better now"). She is tearful in describing the loss of her psychiatrist. She had tried several other psychiatrists in town but says they all were "losers." She is on multiple medications but venlafaxine at 300mg per day "seems to work best of all the antidepressants." Now, however, it seems to be losing effectiveness.

What themes should you be addressing?

_____

_____

_____

_____

_____

_____

22. A guilt-ridden, highly self-critical man believed he deserved to be punished for his wrongdoings. Upon the insistence of his closest friend, he saw a primary-care physician who prescribed an antidepressant. The patient filled the prescription but did not take the pills.

Why not?

_____

_____

_____

_____

_____

_____

23. Soon after his wife divorced him, a 34-year-old man developed panic disorder with agoraphobia. A few years after the divorce he married a woman whose previous husband had for many years been sexually involved with many other women. When she finally found out, she divorced him. The patient trusted only his mother and new wife to be companions for him outside the house. One of them always drove him to work or took him to visit other people. He began a course of pharmacotherapy for his panic disorder and agoraphobia. As he started to improve, his wife became angry, insisting that he abandon this "awful" treatment.

Explain her response.

_____

_____

_____

_____

_____

_____

24. A 16-year-old boy, upon his parents' insistence, went to a psychiatrist for evaluation of depression. He described his parents as "wanting to control him." He could not say "no" to them. He wanted to get out of the house and be on his own. They thought he was depressed. Because he met criteria for major depression, he was started on venlafaxine. At the 2-week follow-up visit he reported that he had stopped the pills and had "faked" the answers to the depression questions.

Why had he "faked" the answers and agreed to take the pills?

_____

_____

_____

_____

_____

_____

25. A 28-year-old woman used cocaine whenever she felt criticized by her boyfriends. She would then break up with them, saying to herself that she was better off without them. During the initial psychiatric evaluation she fit criteria for depression. She was offered medications but only took them for a few days, insisting that she could take care of herself.

Speculate about her expectations of both the pills and intimate relationships.

_____

_____

_____

_____

_____

26. A 35-year-old schizophrenic woman refused to take medications because she was afraid of them. Her mother, with whom she had been very close, began hearing voices when the patient was a child. Her mother was started on antipsychotic medications and became a "walking zombie." She was institutionalized. The patient rarely saw her mother after that. The patient had decided to treat herself "spiritually," but, she was still unable to leave her apartment without her own voices getting stronger and stronger.

Speculate about the reasons she is afraid of medications now.

_____

_____

_____

_____

_____

_____

27. A 28-year-old bipolar woman desperately sought psychopharmacological help. However, after each 2–4-week trial of a successful medication treatment, she experienced a minor side effect (such as feeling a little groggy the next morning) and stopped the medication. After each discontinuation, she returned to the pharmacotherapist, desperately seeking another medication. This pattern also played out in her romantic relationships.

Describe the romantic relationship pattern.

_____

_____

_____

_____

_____

_____

28. A 45-year-old woman with chronic, undifferentiated schizophrenia was able to organize herself sufficiently to competently raise a child with the support of her parents (after Mintz, in press). Unfortunately, her child died of cancer, sending her more deeply into psychosis. Her parents urged her to seek treatment. She accepted medication only when her intense loneliness brought on the friendly voices of her comforting psychosis. However, she developed severe side effects (trembling, nausea, dizziness, difficulty walking due to the medications) and discontinued them, preferring antipsychotics that were ineffective. She was preoccupied with her dead child and the psychotic conviction that she could cure deadly disease and bring back the dead.

Explain her attitude toward medications.

_____

_____

_____

_____

_____

_____

SUGGESTED ANSWERS/COMMENTARY

Inpatient Case

1. The patient may not wish to become pregnant and this may be a source of conflict with her husband—a conflict potentially contributing to her depressed mood. When you subsequently to interview the patient alone, you can use your discussion of medication alternatives to explore her views about becoming pregnant.

Emergency Department Cases

1. The patient may not know how to handle the transition from being a full-time homemaker to beginning to work. She might benefit from further exploration of the meaning of this change to her. The goal of the initial interview would not be to challenge the patient regarding the etiology of her symptoms. You could tell her that her symptoms might indeed be due to a medical etiology. But until something is found, not having a diagnosis may be an additional cause of distress, and the patient might benefit from discussing that with someone. If the patient then agrees to the referral, you might let her psychiatrist know about your suspicions.

2. Align with the patient's grandiosity. Agree that he is special and let him know that the research assistant, who will explain the risks and benefits of the study, would be very interested in speaking with him.

3. You could ask the patient if she is aware that if she wants to have her own children in the future, her body must be at a physically healthy enough weight that ovulation would take place. Attaining a healthy weight now is one of the best ways to preserve the option of childbearing in the future.

Outpatient Cases

1. He failed to consider that stopping the imipramine may have had something to do with the attack. When presented with this possibility, he was surprised by his failure to consider it. He then was able to consider the possibility that he had other blind spots in his life, especially with regard to his marriage. He began to more carefully consider his wife's criticism of him.

2. She lost confidence in the therapist's ability to predict the side effects of phenelzine. Patients very rarely generalize the dietary restriction list to a wide arena of foods.

3. Stopping her medications was a way to break away and indirectly express her anger at his remark. When this transference reaction was described to her, she agreed, did not stop her pills, and apologized at the next visit for her call. She added that she was turning her anger at the psychiatrist against herself. The psychiatrist also apologized for his clumsy, accusatory comment.

4. Stay on the paroxetine indefinitely. There were no clear psychotherapeutic issues to discuss. If she has problems when she faces a life stressor, she should return to therapy to prevent further deterioration and find better ways of responding to such stressors.

5. When she was unable to help someone she loved, she became depressed. She could not save her dying son, her grandchildren, or her probation-breaking son. Three months after restarting treatment she seemed to

recover well. Nine months later she returned for a follow-up visit. She reported having had several "episodes" but handled them. She admitted there were times when she went from bed to couch, did not eat, and did not socialize, but because she recognized their origins, she got over them quickly. This latest frustration was triggered by being unable to help her grandchildren once again. Their aunt who had taken them to visit others in her town, had not brought them to visit her.

She was on p.r.n. clonazepam for sleep and Kava Kava (one pill, with an uncertain percentage of kavalactones in a standardized extract). She was confident that she could handle her responses to future failures to save loved ones. She continued to receive regular medication follow-up visits and agreed to keep a diary of her frustrations and depressive experiences. Writing helped to identify situations in which she was allowing her other two children to take advantage of her. Once she clearly recognized her role in these behaviors, she took steps to change. She became proactive in responding to her failed rescuer pattern, no longer holding herself responsible for events she could not control.

6. He put the needs of others ahead of himself. When the therapist mentioned this, the patient began thinking about the many situations in which he had not requested what he wanted. He realized that he needed to ask his wife to work with him on their relationship.

This intervention appeared to be a turning point for him. Over the next year he began to ask for what he wanted from his wife rather than simply accommodating her. He then requested that she join him in marital therapy. When she refused, he requested divorce proceedings. The divorce was difficult for all concerned, though he felt much clearer about what he wanted. He became involved with another woman. After several months of intense romance, he found himself once again putting his needs second to her need to "find herself." He was able to make his wishes known to her, but she refused to continue seeing him for reasons that were never clear to him. He became even more depressed and accepted a referral for psychotherapy. During those sessions he began to understand much more clearly his longstanding pattern of expecting little for himself, a pattern that long preceded his recent lost love. He unraveled the knot of his ambivalent desire for self-value. At termination he was in a new relationship, one in which he was able to ask that his needs to be acknowledged. She, much to his delight, did so.

7. He wanted to comply with the psychiatrist's expectations, which illustrated his need to comply with the expectations of others even when it hurt him to do so.

8. For her, cocaine and sex were the two ways she could feel worthwhile. Without either one, she felt worthless.

9. Perhaps the patient felt guilty about the many people he had killed. Perhaps, if he let anything or anyone help him, he would have to let down his guard and in this way would become vulnerable.

10. A. An alcoholic may incorrectly believe that the medication will harm his or her liver.

 B. The patient may fear becoming addicted to a prescription drug.

 C. The patient may wish to be the one who chooses which drug to take rather than trusting the advice of another person. For example, the patient may have once accepted a drug that someone had said was not addictive, but actually was.

 D. Taking a prescribed medication may force the person to acknowledge that he or she really does have a problem.

 E. The patient may be in Alcoholics Anonymous, where many members think all drugs are bad.

11. The slow increase in dose was based on systematic desensitization. The comment about side effects utilized paradox.

12. He is optimistic about the possibilities but seems never to give them a sufficient chance. The psychiatrist could

ask: "How long will it take you to decide the medication will not work? When will you tell me about your decision to stop?" Or perhaps the patient is ambivalent about taking medication for various reasons, including loss of control, stigma, or religious beliefs. He might best be engaged in psychotherapy, where he could be helped to better understand how the meaning of medications to him represent a central maladaptive pattern.

13. The psychiatrist e-mailed the patient, followed his symptoms and improvement, and in this way helped to heal the rift caused by his ignorance of the patient's history.

14. He was also anxious with his patients. His anxiety negatively affected his therapeutic alliances. The poor therapeutic alliances contributed to poor outcomes.

15. A. Bad reactions to previous medications.

   B. Wanting to be treated perfectly by others or not at all.

   C. Fear of accepting suggestions from an authority figure.

16. A. He felt better, so why continue?

   B. He did not like to think he had to depend upon pills to feel better.

   C. He did not like the "sick role" that medications put him in.

   D. He felt guilty about feeling better in the absence of his wife.

17. A. Announce termination early, at least 3–6 months ahead of time.

   B. Inform patients that occasionally people have difficulty during the transition.

   C. Request responses from patients about the loss and transition.

   D. Arrange an early meeting with the new psychiatrist, emphasizing the value of a fresh outlook.

E. Consider the potential value of short-term psychotherapy.

F. Consider the use of a standardized protocol (see
Mischoulon et al., 2000).

18. (No answers, just a stimulus for discussion)
19. Two weeks later the patient returned, looking much
better. His mood was improved and his fatigue was
gone. Just as the psychiatrist was about to sing the
praises of modern brain chemistry, the lawyer
explained that he never took the drug. He had
checked with a few trusted colleagues in the firm.
They told him that when he had first joined the firm,
he had aggravated them with his sharp, all-knowing
attitude but that the more open attitude he had developed over that last several years had earned their
respect. It was *his* boss who had become known for
his scathing tongue; rumors suggested that the conflicts were between his boss and the other partners.
He was valued at work, and his job was not in jeop-
ardy.

20. Countertransference possibilities: (1) avoiding intense
emotions, (2) unwillingness to see himself as highly
valued by the patient. Possible patient reactions:
(1) discounted, unimportant, devalued, (2) angry, hurt,
(3) reminded of previous losses in which the other person seemed indifferent to the separation.

21. First, pharmacotherapy is the least of your worries.
Raising the dose of venlafaxine to 450mg should be
considered. But no other medication changes should
be tried until the relationship is solidified. Second,
address the pain of her loss of the previous psychiatrist.
Third, fight through the countertransference of "borderline," multiple psychiatric hospitalizations, and suicide attempts. Fourth, address her fear that she might
not find a psychiatrist with whom she can work while
making clear that each of you have the option to refuse
to work together.

22. He believed he should continue to suffer and did not
deserve to feel good.

23. She feared that he would now be loose on the world and begin sexual involvements with other women like her previous husband. She liked knowing where he was at all times.
24. He did what his parents had asked him to do but then decided that he was not being honest with himself.
25. Like the cocaine, the antidepressants were supposed to make her feel good right away. She also believed her relationships should be instantly better and never have difficulty.
26. The pills might lead her to be institutionalized like her mother. The pills also might cut her off from her spiritual connection.
27. If anything minor went wrong in the relationship, she ended it.
28. If she became nonpsychotic, then her child had died forever. She would then have to experience grief over his loss.

RESPONSES OF PSYCHIATRIC RESIDENTS

What is the major difference between supportive psychotherapy and "change-oriented" psychotherapy? During supportive psychotherapy, the aim is not necessarily to find a pattern to change and then to change it. The trainees found this distinction to be quite useful. Discussion of terminating pharmacotherapy suggested that these relationships are more important than trainees wanted to think. For patients, these terminations can be major losses even though they may see each other only at monthly intervals. Therefore, termination of pharmacotherapy should be addressed similarly to termination of psychotherapy. Vignette #1 of the outpatient cases generated speculation about several causes for the man's panic attack, including a pattern of missing important problems and the dangers of stopping medication simply because the physical symptoms subside. Vignette #2 of the outpatient cases led trainees first to think about resistance and possible transference, but then they began to see that an anxious patient might generalize from one anxiety stimulus to several related ones including other foods and other pills (the birth control pills).

RESIDENTS ASKED

How does a pharmacotherapist discuss potential side effects? Should they all be listed? Some patients go directly to the *Physicians' Desk Reference (PDR)* and scare themselves with all the possibilities. How do therapists make choices about what side effects to describe? The trainees discussed the various attitudes toward giving medications, including being overconfident, confident, realistic, and hesitant. Most critical, they thought, was the patient's expectation. Do they prefer to have many choices? Do they prefer a more directive or a nondirective approach?

We discussed one of the trainee's new bipolar patients. During the first session the trainee raised the patient's lithium dose because the patient was rambling on about his girlfriend. When the patient returned the next time, he felt worse and blamed the therapist. In fact, his girlfriend had asked him to leave their apartment. Trainees learned to consider when increased symptoms might be related to the disorder itself and when they might be due to environmental factors.

CONTINUING RESIDENT RESPONSES

Vignette #3 continued to challenge residents to think about pharmacotherapy as having psychotherapeutic aspects including the patients acting out in pharmacotherapy a transference response to the psychiatrist.

Vignette #4 attempted to demonstrate perhaps the only solid way of defining what medication to give a patient: the history of a family member having a positive response.

Vignette #5 challenged the residents to think of recurrent depression as not simply a kind of biological clock being activated into a depressive time, but rather that recurrent events may trigger recurrent depression. They prefer to consider the patient to be a recurrent depression relying on research to suggest the patient should stay on antidepressants indefinitely because of recurrent episodes. This case challenges them to consider the possibility that adequate psychotherapeutic intervention might be sufficient in preventing the need for ongoing pharmacotherapy.

Vignette #6 was bothersome to the residents. "People are late because they are late," said one of them. As in psychodynamically informed psychotherapy, behavior around the therapeutic contract can illustrate sometimes crucial interpersonal patterns.

Vignette #7 was easy for the residents by now because they could see a longstanding pattern acted out in the pharmacotherapeutic relationship.

Vignette #8 also let them see that it is a person who takes the medication not a diagnosis. People have various reasons for beginning, maintaining, and stopping them. It continued to seem problematic to them that patients were individuals responding individually and sometimes idiosyncratically.

Vignette #10 brought many different responses. The fundamental irony is the drug abuser who doesn't want to take "corporate chemicals," and has many reasons for not wanting to do so. By this time, the residents were becoming convinced that there are special psychological reasons for people to take medications that can help them understand the patients and maybe enhance pharmacotherapeutic response.

Vignette #13 surprised the residents in that the psychiatrist was confused about the medications the patients had been taking. "How could the psychiatrist not know what the patient had been taking?" Then as they looked back on their own brief pharmacotherapeutic experiences, a few noticed that although they might have thought they remembered what was in the chart, what actually was in the chart was different. Now as during psychotherapy when there was a breach in the relationship, the most important objective was to heal that breach.

Vignette #14 reminded the residents of a few colleagues of theirs whose names they did not feel like mentioning. They implicitly and now more explicitly recognized that personality patterns in their social worlds enter into their pharmacotherapeutic world.

Vignette #19 challenged the residents to come up with an alternative outcome that they might not have considered. None guessed it.

Vignette #20 touched their fears and problems around terminating. They had become sensitized to the problems patients have in leaving pharmacotherapy. They also had to become more sensitive to their own responses. The self-depreciating response of the young psychiatrist forced them once again to have to consider the possibility that they were more meaningful to their patients than they would like to think.

The residents found Vignette #23 humorous. The patient was being successfully treated and the wife was angry about it. Even though they understood her reasons for it they still found it hard to believe. This case illustrated the impact on family dynamics of successful pharmacotherapy: sometimes successful pharmacotherapy causes more problems than solutions.

Vignettes #25 and 27 elevated transferential responses to yet a higher level for the residents. Here the patients were relating to the medication in ways that they had related to boyfriends. Could this be possible?

Vignette #28 illustrated once again that being psychotic or in some other dysphoric state may in some way be preferred to being more normal.

A Physician, a Nonmedical Psychotherapist, and a Patient:

The Pharmacotherapy-Psychotherapy Triangle

INTRODUCTION

Although managed care companies have strongly contributed to the creation of the mind-brain split by fostering the idea that psychiatrists "do the pills" and other mental health professionals "do the psychotherapy," these triangles have long been part of the landscape of mental health treatment. A survey of psychologists and psychiatrists done in the early 1980s in the state of Washington suggested that these triangles were quite common. Of the 217 responding psychiatrists, 63% treated at least one pharmacotherapy patient concurrently working with a psychotherapist. Of the psychologists, 79% were seeing patients in psychotherapy who were receiving medications from a physician (Chiles, Carlin, Benjamin, & Beitman, 1991). The percentages and total number of such triangles can only have increased since then. The majority of the increase lies in the greater number of primary-care physicians who send their antidepressant prescribed patients to psychotherapists. Psychiatrists provide approximately 35% of the pharmacotherapy to patients with psychiatric disorders in the United States (Thase, Part II of this book; also see "Challenges of Split Treatment" in Part II).

Several issues require clarification in the initiating and maintaining of these triangles:

1. Does the patient understand and accept that an "envelope of confidentiality" surrounds both professionals? In other words, if something the patient tells one provider might be relevant to the other provider's treatment plan, the first provider is legally permitted to tell the other provider.

2. Will notes be exchanged between the professionals if they are not working off the same chart? For example, some patients exaggerate their symptoms to the psychotherapist and minimize them to the psychiatrist.

3. The referring professional should never commit the other professional to a course of treatment. A patient should never be told he or she will receive medications or psychotherapy.

4. Who is responsible for which emergencies? If the problem involves medication side effects, the physician is primarily responsible. If the problem involves interpersonal difficulties, the psychotherapist is primarily responsible. If the patient is dysphoric, confused, or suicidal, the responsible professional is less clear. In most cases, the patient is able to call either one. If the patient needs hospitalization, the physician is the responsible person. If the psychotherapist leaves town, whom does the patient call—the psychotherapist's colleagues or the psychiatrist? If the psychiatrist leaves town, whom does the patient call?

5. An interesting problem: As couples begin psychotherapy, one of the pair may be defined as having a medication-responsive set of symptoms. A referral for pharmacological evaluation might, in the nonreferred person's mind, invalidate the usefulness of couple's therapy. ("He/she is sick. That's why we are having all these problems.") One solution is to refer both people for pharmacological evaluation so that medications can be discussed in the context of the couple's psychotherapeutic work.

Two general classes of triangles are based upon the nature of the prior relationship between the two professionals. In the Washington survey mentioned earlier (Chiles et al., 1991), the single greatest source of referral was friendship (26%), followed by working for the same agency (21%), working in the same building (16%), and sharing an office (11%). Agency referrals tend to be obligatory; friendship referrals tend to be collegial.

The obligatory referral. Because of the professional limitations of the organization referring professional, or because of the limits of the managed care panel and providers, the referrer has a limited set of options for the other leg of the triangle. Sometimes the two professionals work well together; sometimes they don't. When the professionals do not respect each other, patients can be caught in the animosity. In some managed care plans with large panels of mental health treatment providers, the members of the triangle do not even know each other. Should they? If so, when?

The collegial referral. In this case the referring professional likes and respects the consultant. If there are problems, they can discuss them when they see each other informally; if there is a major problem, they feel comfortable calling each other.

A 1997 survey of 276 patients with mood disorders treated by 193 psychiatrists using both pharmacotherapy and psychotherapy found several variables that influenced whether the patient was treated by a psychiatrist alone or by a psychiatrist and nonmedical psychotherapist. Sixty percent of these patients were treated by a psychiatrist alone. The most crucial variable was whether the patient-doctor relationship was subject to utilization management by a managed care organization. If the relationship was subject to management, the patient was four times more likely to be in split treatment. Bipolar patients were more likely to be in split treatment than those with major depressive disorder (34% versus 18%). Patients with younger psychiatrists (31–43 years old) were more likely to be in split treatment than patients seen by older psychiatrists (44–54) (32% versus 21%) (Duffy, 2001). Mintz (in press) reported that patients seen by the psychiatrist only were 10% more compliant with medications than those seen in split treatment.

Despite the tremendous number of such triangles— estimated at around 270,000 in the United States in the early 1980s (Beitman, Chiles, & Carlin, 1984)—only rarely do clinicians create a formal working relationship with the other provider. Contrary to this finding, Bascue and Zlotowski (1980) reported that only 36% of psychologists whose patients were being seen by a physician for medications did not attempt to work with their patient's prescribing physicians.

Woodward, Duckworth, and Gutheil (1993) recommended that a three-way therapeutic contract be initiated at the time of referral to the second professional. The contract should include: (1) the purpose of each treatment, (2) the clinicians' roles, (3) the frequency, time, place, and fee for visits with each clinician, (4) policies for communication between the clinicians, (5) stipulations about supervision of one clinician by another, (6) whom the patient should call in an emergency, (7) arrangements for coverage outside of regular hours and during absences, (8) and any exceptions to the confidentiality of the written record.

These arrangements vary with practice setting (private versus institutional) and clinicians' administrative relationships (friendly versus hierarchical). At the very least the contract calls into awareness the two different clinical perspectives on treatment: the psychotherapist seeks self-understanding and behavior change while the psychopharmacologist seeks diagnosis and adherence to the medication regimen. The psychotherapist may value some distress in promoting growth; the psychopharmacologist seeks symptom reduction. Conflicts occur. For example, Mintz (in press) reported that psychotherapists who are struggling with patients often seek psychopharmacological "magic" from the psychiatrist. The psychiatrist then feels unsupported because the limits of pharmacotherapy may have been reached.

VIGNETTES

1. **Psychotherapist:** How is your drug treatment going? Are you taking your medication as directed?
    Patient: Well, some of the time.
    Psychotherapist: When don't you take it? What gets in the way?
    Patient: I just forget. I'm supposed to take it once a day.
    Psychotherapist: Sure that happens. There are ways to remember. Any other reasons why you sometimes miss a dose?

Patient: I think I don't feel like having sex anymore and I think the pills have something to do with that. (Chiles et al., 1991, p. 112.)

What should the therapist say?

_____

_____

_____

_____

_____

_____

2.   **Psychiatrist:** How is your psychotherapy going?
     Patient: So-so.
     Psychiatrist: Are you having some difficulty with it?
     Patient: It's Dr. Smith. She seems kind of cold. Not like you. You seem to understand me better.

     What should the psychiatrist say?

_____

_____

_____

_____

_____

_____

3.   A couple had been in psychotherapy with a counselor for several months. During this time, the wife had become increasingly withdrawn. The husband reported that she seemed depressed and was not her "old self." She was referred to a psychopharmacologist for evaluation of depression. She started the session stating the

she was feeling fine and that she was having an affair. Her husband did not know.

What can be done?

_____

_____

_____

_____

_____

_____

4. A regional behavioral health care company has the following policy: Any patient who sees a nonpsychiatrist and fits one of the following diagnostic categories must be seen by a psychiatrist immediately after the initial interview: attention deficit disorder, anxiety disorder, major depression and dysthymia, schizophrenia and other psychotic disorders, bipolar disorder, and eating disorders. The psychiatrists perform 10–15 minutes of medication management and do no formal psychotherapy.

Critically evaluate this policy addressing the question of when it is in the patient's best interest to have the psychiatrist do both pharmacotherapy and psychotherapy.

_____

_____

_____

_____

_____

_____

5. A psychiatrist is able to utilize both pharmacotherapy and psychotherapy when treating patients. In the following situations, for what reasons should the psychiatrist consider splitting the treatment? (1) the initial assessment, (2) a pharmacotherapy patient who, after a period of stabilization, now requires longer sessions focused on psychotherapeutic issues, and (3) pharmacotherapy during psychotherapy.

_____

_____

_____

_____

_____

_____

6. After having seen a 45-year-old mother of three college age students for 3 years, a male psychiatrist thought that he had reached the limits of his ability to help her with psychotherapy and suggested that she be referred to a woman therapist in his clinic. He would continue the pharmacotherapy. She had started therapy after separating from her husband because she believed he did not care about her. No amount of drinking and arguing could get his attention. She moved out on her own and got a new job. The psychiatrist attempted to help the couple to resolve their ambivalence about staying together by meeting with both of them several times. She wanted her husband to understand her need for affection from him. She wanted him to want to change. He, on the other hand, was deeply hurt by her leaving and did not want to change. Although he never said it directly, he seemed to want a divorce. When the divorce came the patient continued to ask for a reunion. This did not occur. After she had settled into a new life, a new job, and seemed modestly stable, the psychiatrist suggested the psychotherapy referral.

The patient saw a woman therapist whom she described as friendly and supportive. The new therapist reported to the psychiatrist that the patient seemed to be doing well. Then, a few days after seeing the new therapist, the patient was told that she had made several minor errors at work. In an uncontrollable rage, she attempted to cut her wrists.

Why?

_____

_____

_____

_____

_____

_____

_____

7. A 29-year-old woman presented with bipolar disorder, PTSD (posttraumatic stress disorder), and borderline character traits (after Mintz, in press). She was living at home, unable to work, sleeping long into the morning, had no motivation, and felt very hopeless. Because the patient had made many bad decisions in her life, her parents feared for her safety in the world and undermined any sense of aliveness or competency she might have felt in order to preserve their mutual dependence. When the patient labeled herself for the psychopharmacologist as "bipolar," she added that the label made her feel less guilty. Successful pharmacotherapy would keep her from feeling any emotions as well as reduce the intensity of mood swings.

What could the psychopharmacologist tell the psychotherapist that might be helpful during psychotherapy with this patient?

_____

_____

_____

_____

_____

8. A patient in split treatment asked his psychiatrist about her marital status and preferences in music. How should the psychiatrist handle these questions?

_____

_____

_____

_____

_____

9. A highly intelligent, very successful professional woman in split treatment was referred to a psychiatrist for medication management after her previous psychiatrist retired. The new psychiatrist has never met the current psychotherapist, who had seen the patient in individual psychotherapy for the past three years. After a few sessions, the psychiatrist discovered that the patient's husband gave her the medications every day. The regimen involved three different medications but was not particularly confusing. In addition, the patient seemed to misunderstand the psychiatrist's medication instructions.

What might have been going on here?

_____

_____

_____

_____

_____

_____

SUGGESTED ANSWERS/COMMENTARY

1. "That may be a side effect of the medication. Please talk with Dr. Jones about the sexual side effects and also about ways to remember to take the medication. I will mention these concerns to him as well."

2. "Psychotherapy can stir up strong emotions. Please consider discussing your feelings with her. It may be hard, but talking about negative feelings often leads to good results in the kind of therapeutic work you are doing. I'll be checking with her in a few weeks. I think you'll be glad you talked over these feelings with her." (This supports the colleague and avoids splitting the two professionals into one good and one bad.)

3. It's hard to say what to do. The psychiatrist needed an agreement with the psychotherapist to be included in the envelope of confidentiality. Perhaps the husband should have been included in the initial psychopharmacological evaluation.

4. Psychiatrists should probably see complicated patients for both pharmacotherapy and psychotherapy to manage the potential interaction among the two treatments. Complicated patients tend to place excessive meaning on medications. However some patients are so difficult that simply having two people help is most preferable. This question needs clearer guidelines

5. Among the many possible answers:

    A. Initial assessment: when the psychiatrist does not feel competent to handle one of the treatments with a specific patient.

    B. With the pharmacotherapy patient: when the psychiatrist believes that the nature of their pharmacotherapy relationship does not permit sufficient flexibility to expand into longer psychotherapy sessions.

C. During combined treatment: when most of the session time is consumed by symptoms apparently responsive to pharmacotherapy but never controlled by multiple medication adjustments so that psychotherapeutic issues are not addressed. Here the psychiatrist might refer to another psychiatrist for pharmacotherapy and keep the psychotherapeutic contract.

6. She had felt rejected by her psychiatrist, just as she had been rejected by her husband. The criticism at work was a small reminder of these two rejections. She returned to her psychiatrist, and asked him to continue seeing her. She was reluctant, however, to discuss the rejection.

7. The patient is attempting to split her treatment along biological lines. If medications keep her quiet and numb it will comfort her parents. That nonfeeling state, however, would prevent her from engaging the world. She needs to examine this desire to use medication to support her family's wish that she remain disengaged from the world.

8. The patient may be attempting to fill the time of their session or extend the session, or simply may be trying to be friendly. The psychiatrist should try to find out if this particular instance of modest boundary-crossing illustrates a key maladaptive pattern that is central to the patient's psychotherapy. If so, the patient and psychotherapist can use it as another example of a pattern in need of change.

9. This professionally successful woman may have been using medications as a way to express her dependency on her husband. The psychiatrist could invite the husband in and perhaps begin couples therapy.

RESIDENT RESPONSES TO SPLIT TREATMENT DISCUSSIONS

Trainees described a case involving a patient, a psychotherapist, and a pharmacotherapist. The patient had been severely troubled, requiring hospitalization almost bimonthly. For the past 6 months she had remained outside the hospital with improving social functioning. As they neared the end of their outpatient year, the psychotherapist told the patient that she was transferring out of the clinic. The patient exclaimed, "Is Dr. X (the once-monthly pharmacotherapist) also leaving?" "Yes," came the reply. A few days later the patient became suicidal and needed hospitalization. As trainees discussed the case they emphasized only the medication "errors." Abandonment probably played a bigger part.

The Sequencing Problem (Using Panic Disorder as an Example)

INTRODUCTION

Research designs comparing pharmacotherapy versus psychotherapy versus the combination (and possibly placebo controls and wait list controls) are prohibitively expensive. So how do we test various sequencing hypotheses—first one, then the other, versus both treatments simultaneously? These studies are even more complex and therefore more expensive. This forces clinicians to base these decisions on a number of sources of information, including but not limited to: patient preference, diagnosis, family history, symptom severity, previous responses to treatment as well as psychiatrist experiences, preference, and intuition. When should family therapy and group therapy become part of the sequence in addition to individual psychotherapy? Other questions include the timing and use of case management, day treatment and group homes. Influencing all of these decisions are not only availability of various treatment options but also the patient's economic resources.

For simplicity, this discussion will narrow the question to decisions regarding individual psychotherapy and pharmacotherapy. Clearly there are a significant number of other variables that research designs will never address.

Diagnosis can help determine the sequence. Some diagnostic problems require medications first: schizophrenia, bipolar disorder, and recurrent major depression. Others require psychotherapy first: simple phobias, unresolved grief, and adjustment reactions. For many disorders, diagnosis does not clearly indicate the optimal sequence: panic disorder, generalized anxiety disorder (GAD), posttramatic stress disorder (PTSD), first episode major depression, dysthymia, substance abuse, and borderline personality disorders (BPD) (Karasu, 1982).

When the clinician is presented with a set of problems for which either psychotherapy or pharmacotherapy or both might be useful, there are several strategic options: (1) prescribe medications and conduct psychotherapy at the outset, (2) sequence or cascade the treatments, and (3) match treatment to patient characteristics (after Miller & Keitner, 1996).

The first strategy, although quite common, may not be cost-effective because some patients respond to fewer or less intensive treatments. It is also possible that combined treatments can, in some situations, be problematic. On the other hand, simultaneous treatments can be synergistic.

The second strategy requires that the patient first be offered one treatment alone. Psychiatrists tend to offer pharmacotherapy first and psychotherapists tend to offer psychotherapy first. If the patient responds, no additional treatment may be necessary. If the patient does not respond, a second treatment can be added or, more rarely, substituted for the first treatment. The sequential model has the advantage of cost-effectiveness and is appealing to clinicians who practice only one treatment approach or who do not have access to other treatment alternatives. On the other hand, the sequential model can delay effective treatment combinations, resulting in a significantly longer period of dysfunction. The longer the course of social and/or work dysfunction, the more difficult the recovery.

The "matching" or "prescriptive" strategy attempts to match particular combinations of treatment to particular patient characteristics. The several varieties of matching include (1) deficit matching, (2) resource matching, (3) severity matching, and (4) patient belief. Unfortunately, specific, well-tested prescriptive algorithms are rare in psychiatric practice.

In "deficit matching," treatments are delivered to address specific weaknesses within the presenting symptom complex. For example, a woman with strong neurovegetative signs of depression and a highly critical husband might be offered an antidepressant medication and couples therapy because spousal criticism is highly correlated with relapse. The "resource matching" approach might build on a patient's predisposition toward rational problem-solving by offering cognitive therapy. "Severity matching" commonly guides treatment selection for depression and anxiety disorders in that more severe disorders are likely to be treated by both medication and psychotherapy. Patient beliefs continuously guide treatment selection: why offer pharmacotherapy to a patient with panic disorder who wants to proceed only with psychotherapy?

A study undertaken by the National Institute of Drug and Alcohol Abuse (Project MATCH Research Group, 1997) involved 1726 patients and matched three psychotherapeutic treatment approaches to alcoholism with a large number of patient characteristics. The three psychotherapeutic approaches were: cognitive behavior therapy, twelve-step facilitation (which uses Alcohol Anonymous ideas and meetings), and motivational enhancement therapy (which increases readiness to change). Unfortunately, remarkably little was found to guide clinical formulation of psychotherapeutic treatment based upon patient characteristics. The main finding was that all three psychotherapies worked. Overall, about 50% of the patients were either abstinent or had significant reductions in alcohol use 1 and 3 years after the 12-week treatment periods. It was found that: (1) those patients with more psychiatric disturbances responded better to CBT than to twelve-step facilitation, (2) those scoring high in anger responded better to motivational enhancement therapy, and (3) those with a social network of heavy drinkers responded better to twelve-step facilitation at long-term follow-up (Project MATCH Research Group, 1997). Despite these limited findings, clinicians seek out those characteristics that might indicate the usefulness of one treatment form over another.

Adding medications to the psychosocial treatment of substance abuse illustrates the remarkable complexity of sequence decision making. Factors involved with timing include: the length of abstinence, target symptoms, the severity and clarity of a co-occurring psychiatric disorder, polysubstance dependence, motivation to change, patient and physician preferences. Medication can be considered to target narrow bands of symptoms while relatively minor variations in psychotherapy are required to adapt psychotherapy approaches to specific substance-use problems. Detoxification for alcohol abuse may require benzodiazepines, whereas many different drugs may be useful during a protracted abstinence (e.g., disulfiram, naltrexone, acamprosate) (Ziedonis, Krejci, & Atdjian, 2001).

Building on the work of Cloninger, Svrakic, and Pryzbeck (1993), Gabbard (2000) outlined a pharmacotherapy and psychotherapy approach to the treatment of personality disorders. Pharmacotherapy, he suggested, could address the relatively fixed, genetically determined "temperament" qualities of personality while psychotherapy could address the more environmentally determined "character" qualities of personality. "Temperament" includes: tendency to seek novelty, harm avoidance, dependence on reward for continuing a behavior, and persistence. These qualities are each independently inherited. "Character" qualities are primarily shaped by environment. They include degrees of self-directedness (ability to be responsible for self) and cooperativeness (self-other relationships). All personality disorders show low scores on these two character dimensions. Although yet to be tested, pharmacotherapy could address the impulsiveness and emotional liability related to inherited temperament whereas psychotherapy could address the more malleable self-directedness and cooperativeness.

Borderline patients present with a spectrum of symptoms that may be differentially responsive to medications. At least five types of borderline patients may present for treatment. On the basis of clinical observations and with some research, these five types—in order of decreasing responsiveness to medications—are: affective, impulsive, aggressive, dependent, and empty. Psychotherapy appears to be generally useful for each type (Oldham, 2001).

Panic Disorder

Tools for the treatment of panic disorder. Clinicians have at their disposal several chemical and psychotherapeutic approaches. Medications include the SSRIs (selective seratonin reuptake inhibitors), the nonSSRIs (e.g., venlafaxine, nefazodone), the tricyclic antidepressants (e.g., imipramine), benzodiazepines, monamine oxidase inhibitors (e.g., phenelzine), and gabapentin. Psychotherapeutic approaches include cognitive therapy and psychodynamic approaches as well as exposure, through desensitization, for the often-accompanying agoraphobia. The psychotherapeutic approaches have in common the identification of phobic stimuli followed by various techniques to address them cognitively, emotionally, and behaviorally. There are seven general phobic stimuli for panic disorder patients:

1. Fear of returning to a place in which a previous panic attack has happened or to another place in which an attack is feared to be likely.
2. Fear of unpleasant body sensations becoming a catastrophic illness (interoceptive phobias) (e.g., chest pain means heart attack).
3. Fear of separation from an important other.
4. Fear of being "suffocated" emotionally by another person.
5. Fear of one's own anger.
6. Activation of a traumatic memory.
7. Activation of unresolved grief.

Identification of the phobic stimulus is facilitated by the cognitive thought record. The patient records cognitions associated with panic attacks while also describing the situation in which the panic attack occurred.

Patient characteristics to be taken into account. Several variables help to narrow the choice of treatments:

1. Does the patient want medications, psychotherapy, both, or is not sure?
2. Is the patient treatment naïve or have there been several unsuccessful/successful treatments?
3. Is there a family history of panic disorder and if so, what worked?
4. How intense are the symptoms now? What degree of agoraphobia is present?
5. What are the comorbid disorders (e.g., major depression, substance abuse)?

6. Are family members interested, involved, and trying to help?

7. What is the payment source (e.g., some managed care companies may not pay for psychotherapy by psychiatrists, so psychotherapy would need to be done by a nonpsychiatrist)?

Psychiatrist variables to be taken into account: How comfortable is the psychiatrist with doing psychotherapy with panic-disorder patients? This comfort varies among psychiatrists.

With these multiple treatment alternatives and patient variables, studying combinations that maximize outcome becomes highly problematic for researchers. Clinicians become "cooks" who mix the ingredients by guidelines and intuition. An algorithm cannot be complete without also being excessively long. Following is an outline for an algorithm for beginning to integrate treatments.

A Panic Disorder Treatment Algorithm

Integrated treatment requires a melding of the sequences of pharmacotherapy with the stages of psychotherapy. The first phase is engagement, which involves making the diagnosis and offering treatment options. This is followed by the initiation of treatment, early maintenance (looking for patterns and early change), and finally the maintenance (change) and possible termination of medications and/or psychotherapy. There are many decision points in each of these stages. The following outline assumes that the psychiatrist is willing and able to do both pharmacotherapy and psychotherapy. Thinking simultaneously in terms of the mind and the brain for panic disorder requires that the psychiatrist not only monitor side effects and symptoms but also continue to search for the potential phobic stimuli triggering the panic attacks. As a reminder, we use the term "integrating" treatments when one person does both pharmacotherapy and psychotherapy although it is quite common to separate the discussion during an interview by focusing at one time only on medications and the other time on psychotherapeutic issues. We use the term "combined" treatment when one person is doing the pharmacotherapy and another doing psychotherapy for the same patient.

To illustrate the implementation of the algorithm, we provide two examples of patients on opposite ends of the severity and treatment-difficulty continuum.

Ms. Z is 30 years old, unmarried, and afraid of men. She has had no previous treatment of any kind, prefers not to take medications, and has no family member or friend directly involved with her problems. She easily used the thought record to define situations in which she panicked. These involved intimacy with men— e.g., doing the dishes with her boyfriend or being on the verge of penetration during sexual activity.

By challenging her own cognitions and past-present interpretations Ms. Z discovered that her fear of men was related to her belief that all men would dominate her as her father had dominated her mother. Her panic attacks were not severe or frequent. She was asked to complete a thought record and began to notice how current anxiety was triggered by thoughts that were not directly relevant to the current situation. After examining a series of thoughts and feelings triggered by a demand her father had made upon her while visiting him at home, she began to see how he attempted to control her. On her next visit to her parents, she started to stand up to him. Her brother was quite surprised at her newfound assertiveness, but not as much as her father was. She broke up with her old boyfriend and started inviting a new man over for dinner regularly. She learned to ask for what she wanted, instead of fearing that any request by her was "being just like my father." She never needed any medications.

Ms. Y presented with depression associated with intense, often intractable nausea that drove her to the emergency department on a regular basis. After a few months it became clear that this nausea was part of a panic disorder. The patient had side effects to all psychoactive medications that she tried. Because of this, she stopped taking them. She refused to think there might be a psychological trigger to these attacks. She formed a positive, intense transference to her psychiatrist. This attachment prevented her from reporting her suicidal ideation, her severe and continuing headaches, and her deepening despair. She did not want him to reject her.

Ms. Y's treatment proceeded very differently, from that of Ms. Z. Her symptoms were frequent and intense. Medications were necessary but she experienced numerous side effects requiring

TABLE 5-1
Integrating Treatments for Panic Disorder*

I. Treatment of Naïve Patient
    A. If the patient wants only medications:
        1. SSRIs, starting at low doses (e.g., paroxetine 10mg, citalopram 10mg, sertraline 25mg) to avoid early pharmacological trigger of panic attacks.
        2. If the patient fears sexual and other side effects of SSRIs, consider a medication such as gabapentin or a benzodiazepine. (The reason to consider gabapentin is its minimal abuse potential and minimal withdrawal symptoms.)
        3. If family member had been successfully treated with pharmacotherapy, consider this medication.
    B. If patient wants only psychotherapy:
        1. Cognitive therapy for interoceptive phobias.
        2. Psychodynamic therapy for anger and/or separation and loss triggers.
        3. Grief work for unresolved grief.
        4. Exposure for traumatic memory.
    C. If not sure what to select:
        1. Psychotherapy or SSRI depending on clinician's predisposition, unless the symptoms are too intense for the patient to tolerate for any extended period, in which case gabapentin or benzodiazepines should be considered.
    D. With agoraphobia:
        1. Systematic exposure (if a significant other is available, he or she facilitates exposure).
    E. With major depression:
        1. Antidepressant, unless the depression is secondary to the panic disorder (i.e., if the patient states, "If the panic goes away, I will not be depressed").
        2. Psychotherapy focused on depressive cognitions and relationship models (include depressive reactions in thought record).
    F. With alcoholism:
        1. Gabapentin or SSRIs (avoid benzodiazepines), recommend AA, and include situations in which drinking occurs as part of the thought record.

Rollman & Shear, personal communication, April 12, 2001.

II.   Treatment of Patients Who Have Undergone Previous Treatment
  A.   Was previous psychotherapy helpful? In what ways? If not helpful, for what reasons? no focus on potential triggers of attacks? problem with the therapeutic relationship?
  B.   If previous medication treatments have been used:
    1.   If "inadequate" SSRI trial (6 weeks at maximum dose), then try an SSRI.
    2.   If positive response to antidepressant, restart the same one.
    3.   If positive response to BZD, recommend beginning with SSRI to see if it is effective before beginning a BZD.
    4.   If intolerant to SSRI consider another one of a different class (e.g., venlafaxine).
III.   Initial Treatment
  A.   Monitor side effects (with SSRIs/TCAs anticipate possible panic attacks in the first week or two).
  B.   Examine potential reasons for stopping medications:
    1.   Consider fear of loss of control, as loss of control is a major fear of panic disorder patients.
    2.   Attempt to relate resistance to medication to triggers for panic attacks.
    3.   Anticipate side effects or lack of immediate responsiveness as potential threats to working alliance. Anticipate that panic patients who are somatically focused are very likely to report even minor side effects.
    4.   Assign thought record homework, being careful to insist that if the patient does not complete it, the therapist will not be critical. Many panic patients are highly sensitive to criticism (e.g., fearing rejection and anger). Failure to complete homework can also be used to examine cognitions.
  C.   With sleeping problems, consider low-dose, sedating antidepressants.Consider amitriptyline (Elavil), doxepin (Sinequan), and trazodone at low bedtime doses. If used with the SSRIs, paroxetine and fluoxetine are more likely than sertraline to increase levels of TCAs due to cytochrome P450 2D6 inhibition. Effective pharmacotherapy can help strengthen the working alliance.

IV.   Looking for Patterns and Beginning of Change/Early Medication Maintenance

    A. Monitor symptoms and side effects:

        1. If partial response, raise doses by 10mg on biweekly basis (e.g., paroxetine from 10mg to 40mg depending upon ability to tolerate and symptoms; some patients may require 60mg).

        2. Consider adding BZD or gabapentin if unable to tolerate current symptoms.

        3. If unable to tolerate SSRIs, begin low-dose nonSSRI (e.g., 37.5mg venlafaxine).

    B. Utilize thought record and other means to identify panic triggers. Explore interpersonal effects of panic attacks (e.g., effects on spouse, parents; effective treatment of panic disorder occasionally leads to divorce, as the major function of the spouse was to help with panic and agoraphobic fears).

    C. For agoraphobics, continue to encourage facing fears in slow, systematic ways, and utilize significant others.

V.   Psychotherapeutic Change/Medication Maintenance

    A. Monitor adherence to medications:

        1. If sexual side effects, develop strategies to counteract.

        2. If on BZD and SSRI/TCA attempt to taper BZD.

    B. Explore the triggers for panic attacks:

        1. Somatic phobias ("Do you really believe you are having a heart attack?").

        2. Anger (origins and fears of expression; learning assertiveness—being neither to passive nor too explosive with anger expression).

        3. Separation anxiety (difficulty in being alone).

        4. PTSD (reexperience traumatic events in safe therapeutic relationship).

        5. Unresolved grief (attempt to let go of the past)

VI.   Termination/Discontinuance of medications

    A. Continue medications for at least 6 months.

        1. Begin discontinuation:
            If symptoms of anticipatory anxiety, phobic avoidance, and panic are remitted.
            If there is no major psychosocial stress.
            If there is no major medical illness.

        2. May discontinue psychotherapy but continue monthly medication visits.

        3. May discontinue both pharmacotherapy and psychotherapy (look for problems in separation, including return of symptoms.)

much psychopharmacological experimenting until moderate levels of benzodiazepines partially helped her anxiety but did little for depression. She was unwilling to discuss her intense transference reaction. Her pathway through the algorithm required integrated and then split treatment. She continued to refuse to discuss psychological issues. She became pregnant and gave birth to a son. Gradually the demands of motherhood forced her to consider the impact of her anxiety on her son. Her psychiatrist felt frustrated with his inability to help and suggested she seek a different psychotherapist. She angrily found another person from the phonebook who did not work out. Her internist began her on amitriptyline 25mg for headaches, which gave her some relief. Seizing upon this amitriptyline surprise (she could tolerate its minor side effects), the psychiatrist raised the dose to reduce her nausea, anxiety, and depression. When the dose was raised the patient finally admitted her suicidal thinking and agreed to see another therapist. Grudgingly she began to acknowledge the terror her mother had instilled in her when she threatened to abandon Ms. Y unless she did exactly what her mother demanded. Her rage was deep and frightening. Courageously, she faced this terror with the help of the new therapist; the psychiatrist remained the encouraging psychopharmacologist. Over the next 2 years improvement gradually continued with many small regressions and medication modifications.

VIGNETTES

1. Lois was a 39-year-old social worker who had been suffering from panic attacks for almost 25 years. She described her first panic attack as follows: "I had my first panic attack when I was 14 years old, and I remember it very clearly. It was in algebra class, and I had done fine—I had always been a good student. There were no particular problems. I don't recall feeling particularly stressed. In the middle of class, I heard a sound. It sounded like it was right behind me, and it was very loud, like a gunshot or an explosion. It startled me very badly. My heart pounded, I was short of breath, and I started shaking. I remember looking around to figure out where the sound came from, but no one else

seemed to have heard anything. That was my first panic attack. My hands shook, my heart pounded, I was short of breath, I was near tears, I had trouble focusing my eyes, and this probably lasted almost 20 minutes. I didn't know what it was. In a very short period of time, I started having panic attacks like that, which would last anywhere from 5 minutes to 20 or 30 minutes. For the next few years, I would have them anywhere from 10 to 20 times a day."

How would you treat her? Psychotherapy? Pharmacotherapy? Both?

_____

_____

_____

_____

_____

_____

2. Lois continued to describe the progression of her panic disorder including social influences:

Lois: I had no language to describe what was happening to me. I was scared to death. The best way that I could describe it to people was to say, "I'm so nervous, I'm so terribly nervous." So my parents took me to our family doctor, who ran some tests but couldn't find anything wrong. I continued to have the problem. I was then referred to a psychiatrist. I recall being put on thioridazine (Mellaril). I remember watching the autumn of 1970 from a rocking chair in the living room. I remember just looking at the trees, watching the leaves change colors. I was a zombie. I could barely move. I could barely function. I could barely think. And everyone was very happy because I suddenly wasn't nervous anymore.

Therapist: You just weren't functioning.

Lois: I wasn't functioning at all. I still had the sensation that there was something terribly wrong, and I knew that the thioridazine was not making it better.

Therapist: So you stayed on the thioridazine for what, about 6 months?

Lois: I stayed on the thioridazine for probably between 3–6 months. I can't remember exactly how long it was.

Therapist: And, how did you get off of it?

Lois: I lied. I pretended to take it, and I stopped taking it. My parents would have had a fit if they had known I had stopped taking it, and I started to function a little bit better, but I continued to have the panic attacks. I was terrified to go back to the psychiatrist because I didn't want to be put back on that medication. Medical doctors—basically everybody—were telling me there was nothing wrong with me physically. I didn't quite know how to handle it. At one point, I was very despondent. I do not truly believe that I was suicidal, but I remember saying something to my mother about how I did not want to live if I had to live like this. It upset my mother very much. My parents sat me down that night and said, "We have taken you to doctors. We have done everything we can, and you're not getting better, and what you have to do is you have to stop telling people about this. You have to stop talking about this because if you don't you will be put away."

With this additional information, design a new treatment plan of pharmacotherapy and/or psychotherapy for Lois.

_____

_____

_____

_____

_____

_____

3.   Later in the session, Lois described her responses to the current pharmacological treatment plan.

Lois: Well, the miracle drug clonazepam at the lowest dose felt really fine. I know one of the side effects is drowsiness and some sedation. I felt no sedation. I felt very energized. I felt really good. And I did notice a decrease in my panic attacks. I did feel a little better regarding the agoraphobia which I haven't really described, but after 24 years of panic attacks I have some pretty strong agoraphobic behaviors—and I had noticed some improvement in that. When we increased the dosage, I had an incident.

Therapist: The dosage was .5mg twice a day.

Lois: Um-hum.

Therapist: And then we went up to 1mg twice a day.

Lois: Um-hum. I picked up my daughter from school one day, and as I was driving her home she told me that some little boy on the playground had been beating up on her. She is 5 years old. I was very upset about that, but she said she was okay and didn't seem particularly disturbed by it. She didn't want me to talk to her teacher or anything, and I had asked her what she had done when this little boy was beating up on her, because I had taught my daughter that if somebody was picking on her or if somebody was hurting her to tell her teacher or an adult that she trusted and they would protect her. I said, "What did you do?" She said she told her teacher and the teacher said just go back out there and hit him back. Well, I was a little miffed because that's not how I'm teaching my daughter to handle things, but she didn't want me to pursue it anymore and I sort of let it go. Somehow, then, over the ensuing 24 to 48 hours I started obsessing about that. I could not get that out of my mind.

Therapist: Couldn't get what out of your mind?

Lois: The fact that somebody was hitting my child. It just boggled my mind. I grew up getting beat up on. I had sworn before I ever had children that that was not going to be them. That I would not hit my children. They would know that there was an adult in this world who loved them who would not hurt them. And, I guess I saw it—I had tried so hard to protect my child from being hurt physically, and I couldn't do it. There were people and things out there that were going to hurt her. I remember having a telephone conversation with my mother during this period when I was obsessing about this, and my mother was laughing it off. She said, "Well, it's about time she learned that this is what the world is like." I got very upset and I thought, you know, my parents didn't feel any particular concern about my being beat up by them or being beat up by my brothers or by a boyfriend. To them, that's the way the world is.

Therapist: Get used to it.

Lois: Get used to it. And, "It's about time your daughter got used to it too." And, it's like something snapped. I had this very strong sense for about 24 hours that I could trust no one to protect my child except me. I came very close to taking her out of school, to quitting my job to stay home and protect her, physically protect her. I had decided I was not going to let my parents see her anymore because they could not be trusted to protect her. I got irrational, and I remember thinking the world is a very evil and scary place and I am the only one that can protect my daughter. And, at that point I thought I must get a gun because that is the only way to protect my child. I remembered thinking, "Where do I get a gun? Why I don't know where to get a gun?" and then I realized that it's because I don't own a gun—you know, I've always been an advocate of gun control, and that's when I realized that my thinking was a little bit irrational, and that's when I called you and said I have a real problem here. And you told me it could be from the clonazepam, and we rapidly decreased the dose, and within about 48 hours I was back feeling fine.

What clues to the psychological triggers of her panic disorder are revealed in this reaction to clonazepam?

_____

_____

_____

_____

_____

_____

4.   **Therapist:** So what effect did your awareness of these paranoid thoughts—which were probably related to your upbringing and current relationships with your parents—have? What effect did they have on your thinking about your panic and your personal life in general?

Lois: Well, I think one of the things that was enlightening for me was that I really believe that now, in retrospect, I can see that I was raised to believe that the world was really a very frightening place. If there was any sort of abuse or bad relationships we experienced within the family, it was always communicated that your family is all you have because no matter how bad it is in the family, it's ten times worse out there. Most of our social connections when I was growing up were extended family. We were sort of a closed family in the sense that we didn't participate in a whole lot of activities and stuff outside of the family. Very religious, hyperreligious upbringing.

Therapist: And very closed boundaries around the family.

Lois: Very closed boundaries. Except for my generation in the family, really no one else has social contacts outside of the extended family. So, it was hard to know when I was growing up how unusual this whole thing was because this was what I was raised with.

Therapist: You told me a story about one of your cousins who went to a famous institution and became a . . .

Lois: Yes, oh, yes. We call that cousin "the one that got away." When he graduated from high school he was accepted at Yale. I was very excited for him. He is a few years younger than I am. The family was absolutely horrified, absolutely livid. They couldn't believe that he would go all the way to Yale just for a college education when he could get it here in the local community. He got his bachelor's degree, got his master's and Ph.D., I think from MIT, and then was a professor at Stanford, and he has never been back.

Therapist: He's never been back?

Lois: No. He got away.

Therapist: That illustrates some of the ways your family operated.

Lois: Um-hum. There is a sense that you're being disloyal if you leave. There is also a sense because of sort of hyperreligious undercurrents going on that the world "out there" is much too full of satanic influences and, you know, it's evil "out there," meaning outside of the church, outside of the family.

Therapist: And I had the feeling that your clonazepam experience helped elucidate what you've just said to yourself.

Lois: I think I realized, too, that it in trying very, very hard to protect my daughter, perhaps I was being the protector that I had always wished I had and had never had. There had never been anyone that I could turn to when I was younger for physical protection or from protection from this terrible panic disorder. No one that I felt I could trust who really had my best interests in mind and I could count on to help me through it. And I think I wanted to be that kind of person for my daughter.

Therapist: Yeah, that's real clear. I mean, that's even clearer than when you've said it before. How has your life been changing now with your awareness of how your family and you have been and still are?

Lois: It has been freeing in a number of respects for me because I have been able to see some areas in my life where I have gotten stuck, and I can't move forward with my life because I have one foot in the role that they expected me to stay in. My family is not real supportive of my getting treatment for this. I have discussed it with a few of them, and my younger brother is fairly supportive. He has symptoms of panic disorder of his own, and he sort of understands it and can acknowledge it. My mother and the rest of the family seem to be like, "Oh, there's nothing wrong with you. There's nothing wrong. Don't say there is anything wrong with you." They have the old-fashioned view of mental illness: there's well and there's sick, and there's nothing in between.

Therapist: Yeah.

Lois: So, I don't really discuss it with them too much. I've been on the paroxetine for 5 months since the Klonopin scare. Since then, I have a fewer panic attacks. The ones that I do have are really very brief, just a few seconds in duration. They don't scare me that much because I sort of know, that it is just a physiologic rush and it's going to pass over me in a few minutes. Right now what I'm really working on is some of the agoraphobia behaviors, and this is going very slowly for me. It is very frustrating. Many things are difficult for me—driving, bridges, sometimes elevators, public speaking, crowds, and the whole list, and I have been making small steps forward, and I try very hard not to get frustrated at not making faster progress.

Follow-up note: Three years later she flew to Australia several times. She has been maintained on 5mg of paroxetine.

SUGGESTED ANSWERS/COMMENTARY

1. If she still has panic attacks with this frequency, she might need BZD right away. Otherwise, they may be severe and chronic enough to begin an SSRI.

2. May need to be careful about suggesting medications because she had such difficulty with the first one. Be clear about what she wants from medications and what psychotherapy might offer. Problem is potentially treatable by either or both approaches.

3. Rage at her parents, fear of being unprotected and alone. Clonazepam disinhibited her. She was excessively reactive to other medications also. For example, with sertraline 25mg, she became numb and reported many strange visual and sensory experiences.

RESIDENT RESPONSES TO PANIC ALGORITHM CASE

This exercise seemed closer to the real world of clinical practice. Trainees debated validity of the benzodiazepine disinhibition phenomenon and its relative value to the patient's change. They had trouble first believing in the idea of disinhibition. Some related it to alcohol's similar effects. Then, to believe that the content of the disinhibition actually had psychotherapeutic relevance became a subject of heated debate.

Briefly Toward a Neurobiology of Psychotherapy

INTRODUCTION

Pharmacotherapy and psychotherapy each in their own way alters brain function. They appear dichotomous because we use different languages to describe their actions. Clinicians seek metaphors to help them cross this linguistic mind-brain barrier. The metaphors must use both neurobiological and mental terms in order to embrace both pharmacotherapy and psychotherapy. Under the assumption that the brain supports mental function in the way that the heart supports blood circulation, the basic target of change is the brain. The effects of psychotherapy on brain function are further developed in Part II in "Psychodynamic Neurobiology."

The term *circuits* may provide a useful metaphor to link mind and brain. Functional neuroanatomists are increasingly focusing upon sets of interacting circuits (Alexander, DeLong, & Strick, 1986) as a way to understand brain function. Anxiety patients are easily able to report recurrent patterns of anxious thought that circle through their consciousness. Psychotherapy's effect on anxiety circuits appears to help patients "step back further" from their anxious thoughts; pharmacotherapy seems to diminish the intensity of these thoughts. Just what these different phrases actually mean in terms of brain function remains speculative.

In order to begin the construction of a model of psychotherapy that can be mapped onto brain function, psychotherapy must be defined in clear, operational terms that offer the possibility of finding a set of brain correlates. Brain function can be divided into three large interacting components: intracellular, intercellular (synapses and circuits), and gross anatomic (e.g., prefrontal cortex, amygdala). Aspects of the brain that are likely to provide the foci and conduits of psychotherapeutic change must be identified if psychotherapeutic processes are to be hypothetically linked to brain processes. Subsequently, increasingly sophisticated information about pharmacological actions must be linked to psychotherapeutic effects if we are to begin to comprehend the summation of the individual effects of pharmacotherapy and psychotherapy. This will then lead to a conceptual and practical integration of mind-brain treatments.

Table 6.1 presents the basic processes of psychotherapeutic change that need to be correlated with brain function. Following each of the processes is a crude attempt to link them to brain function—largely to gross anatomical subdivisions. Note that these processes are taking place not only in the patient's brain but also in the therapist's.

For panic disorder and other diagnostic problems, we clinicians would ideally have a picture in our minds for the targets of our clinical efforts. Some "foggy" images are emerging from neuroscience research for panic disorder (Gorman, Kent, Sullivan, & Coplan, 2000). Following is a simple model involving the prefrontal cortex, the amygdala, and the raphe nuclei:

A hypermetabolic amygdala can be assumed to be a crucial part of the panic/anxiety circuit. We also assume that the projections from the serotonin-containing raphe nuclei "calm" an excited amygdala through serotonin reuptake inhibition. It is also assumed that projections from the prefrontal cortex to the amygdala can have a calming effect as well, being consciously activated.

How does psychotherapy change the way in which patients represent their relationships to other people? These representations are usually unconscious, continuously being built and reformed through the accumulation of multiple interpersonal experiences and utilized in current situations—most often without

TABLE 6-1
Psychotherapeutic Change Processes and Brain Function

Relationship

Empathy: Amygdala (Dicks, Myers, & Kling, 1969; Kluver & Bucy, 1937; Nahm, Damasio, Tranel, & Damasio, 1993; Tranel & Hyman, 1990).
Self-other Representations: Prefrontal cortex-hippocampus (Baron-Cohen et al., 1994; Fletcher et al., 1995).
Social Influence: Serotonin (Yeh, Fricke, & Edwards, 1996).
Self-observation: Frontal–parietal (Duffy & Campbell, 1994).
Readiness to change: Possibly anterior cingulate and prefrontal cortex (suggested in Damasio, 1994)

Defining Patterns

Neurotic Patterns/Circuits: Caudate-prefrontal cortex for obsessive-compulsive disorder (Schwartz, Stoessel, Baxter, Martin, & Phelps, 1996).
Deciding, Choosing, Initiating Change: Ventro-medial prefrontal cortex; basal ganglia (Damasio, 1994; Duffy & Campbell, 1994).
Learning: Synaptic adaptations (Kandel, 1998).
Affect Regulation: Prefrontal cortex-amygdala (Bradley, 2000).

awareness. Neurobiological predispositions and early caregiver interaction patterns lay the groundwork for these self-other representations. These unconscious representations are laid down in what is known as procedural memory.

According to cognitive neuroscience, procedural knowledge is unconscious and becomes inefficient when expressed in verbal terms or made conscious. Its learning takes place in two basic modalities. The first occurs whenever the goals of a new and an older procedure conflict, which requires the deliberate enactment of the new procedure and the active suppression of the older one. Initially the new procedure is inefficient, and the older one may be intrusively enacted. Eventually, both the enactment of the new procedure and the suppression of the old one become fully automatic. This insight mediated process requires time and motivation. These requirements increase sharply in the case of procedures that involve strong emotions.

The second type of learning is not insight mediated. It results from repeatedly observing a procedure being enacted by someone else. This process has not been fully characterized, and its mechanism is poorly understood. This procedural learning is facilitated by a relationship characterized by genuineness and reciprocity, in which negative aspects of the other are not massively disavowed or negated. (Sciolla, 2001, p. 13)

Do medications alter self-other representations and if so, how? How does talking change procedural memory representations of interpersonal relationships? These are questions for the future neurobiology of psychotherapy.

RESIDENT RESPONSES

Some residents protested vigorously against the idea of a "mechanical mind." To think of mind as "only brain" seemed to rob human brains of their humanity. "We are not robots. We have souls," they said. Others argued that improved knowledge of brain function would help our minds function better and perhaps help us to sharpen the distinction between mind and soul

PART II

Research Perspectives, Split Treatment, and Psychodynamic Neurobiology

Conceptual and Empirical Basis for Integrating Psychotherapy and Pharmacotherapy

Michael E. Thase, M.D.[*]

Here we discuss in greater detail than in Section 1 the conceptual and empirical basis for treatment plans that combine medication and psychotherapy. Psychotherapy-pharmacotherapy combinations, hereafter referred to as "combined treatments," generally receive high marks from consumers (Seligman, 1995). They are also often recommended by the expert consensus panels for treatment of specific *DSM-IV* mental disorders (e.g., American Psychiatric Association, 1993, 1997a, 1998; Ballenger, et al., 1998; Depression Guidelines Panel, 1993). It is thus important for mental health professionals to know both the evidence base pertaining to and the indications for combined treatment.

At the beginning of the twenty-first century, concerns about the cost-effectiveness of various interventions are dominant. The costs of providing combined treatment are generally greater during the first 6–12 weeks than those of psychotherapy or pharmacotherapy alone. It also is not practical to treat everyone with both modalities: if combined treatment were provided to everyone seeking mental health care it would overwhelm the capacities of existing health

[*] From the Department of Psychiatry, University of Pittsburgh Medical Center, Western Psychiatric Institute and Clinic, Pittsburgh, Pennsylvania. Please direct all correspondence to Dr. Thase at Western Psychiatric Institute and Clinic, 3811 O'Hara Street, Pittsburgh, Pennsylvania 15213-2593.

services. Thus, there is a great need to demonstrate that combined treatment is superior to either component monotherapy before that approach can be routinely recommended.

In some areas, research evidence from comparative studies does not establish the superiority of combined treatment. Before we assume that such studies have yielded negative data (as opposed to "failed" or false negative results), an evaluation of the research methodologies must be done to ensure the validity of the findings. Specifically, we will examine earlier studies, aided by recent advances in the understanding of clinical trial design and statistical methods. Ultimately, this review will reveal a systematic underestimation of the additive effects of combined treatment, especially among subgroups with more severe mental disorders.

THE RATIONALE FOR PSYCHOTHERAPY-PHARMACOTHERAPY COMBINATIONS

Combined treatment is preferred by a large proportion of mental health professionals. Nevertheless, there has been a persistent concern that symptom-reducing effects of medication might decrease a patient's motivation for gaining insight or making interpersonal or lifestyle changes that might facilitate a sustainable "cure" (see the discussion by Klerman et al., 1994).

There has also been a decades-long debate among psychodynamically oriented therapists about the effect of prescribing medication on the therapeutic relationship. Some propose that a prescribing therapist could be seen as authoritarian or dictatorial. Others suggest that therapists who are unwilling to write prescriptions might be viewed as withholding or even sadistic. If transference is considered to be the prime vehicle for successful psychotherapy, then the intrusion of medical monitoring into the therapeutic relationship may be viewed as distracting.

As evidence demonstrating that various pharmacotherapies were effective treatments for severe mental disorders such as schizophrenia, psychotic depression, bipolar disorder, and obsessive-compulsive disorder continued to emerge in the 1960s and 1970s, use of medications began to be viewed more favorably, specifically as a means to hasten recovery and facilitate progress in psychotherapy (Klerman et al., 1994). Concerns about negative effects dissipated, as there was no evidence of subtractive interactions in the first wave of studies on combined treatment (see Rounsaville, Klerman, & Weissman, 1981). Notably, in the initial studies of schizophrenia, psychotherapy was ineffective unless combined with antipsychotic pharmacotherapy (Hogarty, Ulrich, Mussare, & Aristigueta, 1976; May, 1968). Subsequently, psychotherapy alone was viewed as ineffective for any form of psychosis, including mania and psychotic depression.

Pharmacotherapy alone, however, did not address psychotic patients' underlying vulnerabilities. Even when medication was effective, patients often had persistent interpersonal and vocational difficulties, as well as poor problem-solving skills. Combined treatment thus came to be viewed as the means of lessening psychosocial dysfunction and of improving quality of life over and above the effect of medication alone on core psychotic symptoms. It also was hoped that additional symptomatic relief might emerge over time as a consequence of improved morale, more effective coping with adversity, or reduced sensitivity to day-to-day problems. Psychotherapy also was hoped to have a favorable effect on adherence to medication. Combined treatment thus was presumed to be the best way to broaden the breadth and increase the magnitude of treatment efficacy.

There is also evidence to indicate that at least some forms of psychotherapy, used alone, were useful treatments for anxiety and (nonpsychotic) depressive disorders. Most experts and clinicians presumed that psychotherapy and pharmacotherapy work via non-overlapping mechanisms, which might permit truly additive effects (i.e., 0.5 + 0.5 = 1.0). Indeed, synergistic interactions between treatments might even be possible (i.e., 0.5 + 0.5 = 1.2). Regrettably, synergy has not been evident in studies of combined treatment (Thase, 2000). In fact, the greatest additive effect observed in a study of combined treatment was still rather modest (i.e., 0.5 + 0.5 = 0.8) (Keller et al., 2000). We will refer to this as incomplete summation of therapeutic effects. It is now known that there are both statistical and pragmatic reasons for the failure to demonstrate synergistic or fully additive effects.

One reason for incomplete summation is a methodological artifact known as a "ceiling effect." This refers to a progressive loss of a scale's sensitivity to detect change as the degree of symptomatic improvement increases over time. The scales used to measure outcomes assess symptom severity, rather than indicators of wellness (e.g., mirth, equanimity, flexibility, reciprocity, or patience). Without assessing correlates of superior functioning, it will be difficult to distinguish between the higher grades of response.

Another ceiling effect results when studies include a proportion of sizable treatment-resistant cases. In studies of mood disorders, for example, approximately 10–20% of a typical study group will not respond to any form of treatment (Keller & Boland, 1998; Thase, 2002). In studies of schizophrenia, for example, 50% of a typical study group will not be medication-responsive (American Psychiatric Association, 1999; 2002). Treatment-resistant patients will typically manifest high symptom scores across the trial that inflate both the means and the standard deviations of the outcome measures. To illustrate, the standard deviations of outcome measures such as the Hamilton (HAM-D; Hamilton, 1960) or Beck (BDI; Beck, Ward, Mendelson, Mack, & Erbaugh, 1961) depression rating scales, the Young Mania Rating Scale (YMRS; Young, Biggs, Siegler, & Meyer, 1978), or the Brief Psychiatric Rating Scale (BPRS; Overall & Gorham, 1961) typically double over the course of therapy in randomized controlled trails (RCTs). This reduces the ability to detect small-to-moderate differences in symptom ratings, which decreases the power or design sensitivity of a study.

Distortions of statistical measures of variability also are caused by several common conventions used to analyze the data of patients who drop out of RCTs. This is hardly a trivial matter: Between 10% and 40% of the participants of RCTs drop out before contributing data on their outcomes. One means of compensating for this is employment of the last observation carried forward (LOCF) method, in which the final assessment of the participant is used to impute the outcome. Although this type of "intent-to-treat" (ITT) approach is preferred over a comparison of only those who completed a treatment protocol, the assumption that dropouts would have the same high scores across multiple time points can grossly distort the pattern of scores. Even those who are not responding to a treatment generally feel better as time passes.

A second factor for incomplete summation is the failure to appreciate the magnitude of the effects of so-called common, or nonspecific elements, of helping relationships (Thase, 2002). These effects are typically minimized by use of the term *placebo*

(PBO) *effect*, which does not take into account the critical elements of prognosis (i.e., spontaneous remission), hope/expectation, and the doctor-patient relationship (or therapeutic alliance). In RCTs of antidepressant medications, for example, PBO effects now account for about 75% of the response to pharmacotherapy (Khan, Warner, & Brown, 2000; Thase, 1999). These nonspecific effects similarly account for a majority of the "action" of the depression-focused therapies (Elkin et al., 1989; Jacobson et al., 1996; Krupnick et al., 1996).

The nature of the PBO actually has very little to do with overall response to various kinds of sham treatments in studies of psychiatric disorder (Hrobjartsson & Gotzsche, 2001). In one RCT, a measure of the strength of the helping alliance was as predictive of success in pharmacotherapy (with either imipramine *or* placebo), as it was with cognitive and interpersonal psychotherapies (Krupnick et al., 1996).

Appreciation of the magnitude of nonspecific effects and ceiling effects permits fresh interpretation of existing studies of combined treatment. Using a large study of combined treatment in chronic depression as an example, the left panel of Figure 1 illustrates an apparent "incomplete summation." However, after taking into account the design considerations previously discussed, a fully additive effect or even synergy was observed (see right panel). If it is assumed that approximately 30% of this study group would have responded to a PBO-expectancy intervention (see, for example, Ravindran et al., 1999; Thase, Fava, Halbreich, Kocsis, & Koran, 1996), the "active" components of pharmacotherapy and psychotherapy each delivered a response rate of approximately 20%. Thus, a full addition of therapeutic effects should have resulted in a 70% ITT response rate (i.e., 30% + 20% + 20%); a 72% ITT (intent-to-treat) response rate actually was observed.

It is critical when designing new studies to ensure that enough patients are enrolled to have the statistical power necessary to reliably detect the small-to-modest differences. If a 15% difference in response or remission rates is anticipated, then at least 250 patients will need to be enrolled in *each arm of the* study (Kraemer & Thiemann, 1987). If a difference of greater than 10% is anticipated (i.e., partial summation), then at least 500 patients will need to be enrolled in each arm (see Thase, Entsuah, & Rudolph, 2001).

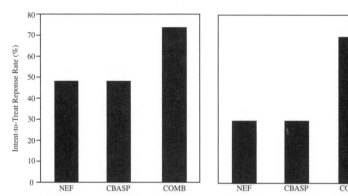

FIGURE 1 Left Panel: The apparent additive effects of the cognitive behavior analysis system of psychotherapy (CBASP) and nefazodone were large (52% relative advantage) in one study of chronic depression, but did not approach a full summation of the benefits of the monotherapies. Right Panel: Removal of the common response rate to placebo-expectancy factors (estimated here as a 30% response rate) reveals a fully additive and possibly synergistic effect for combined treatment (139% relative advantage). (Adapted from Keller et al., 2000.)

The assumption that psychotherapy and pharmacotherapy have different mechanisms of action provides another rationale for the combination treatments. This "shotgun" approach also might be viewed as a two-stage strategy: 1) relatively rapid pharmacologic alleviation of patients' suffering, followed by 2) slower psychotherapeutic gains in social functioning and vulnerability.

An opposite pattern of additive effects has been observed when the outcome moderator is drawn from the psychosocial domain.* Miller, Norman, and Keitner (1990) reported that an overall modest additive effect for the combination of pharmacotherapy and cognitive behavior therapy actually was the average of two distinctly different response profiles. Among the subgroup of patients with elevated levels of dysfunctional attitudes, the combined treatment group was markedly more effective than medication management. By contrast, no such additive effect was observed among the subgroup with more normal levels of dysfunctional cognitions (Figure 2; Miller et al., 1990).

---

* *"A moderator tells for whom or under what conditions a treatment has an effect"* (Kraemer, 200).

Combination treatments also may target specific functional deficits associated with chronic mental disorders, rather than syndromal signs or symptoms. In these cases, the addition of a psychosocial intervention may not result in greater improvement in core psychotic or manic symptoms, but may aid in rehabilitation or enhance longer term psychosocial outcomes.

Psychotherapy can also be aimed at improving medication adherence and might even result in use of lower dosages of medication (e.g., Hersen, Bellack, Himmelhoch, & Thase, 1984). Such effects would translate into cost savings that might help to offset the cost of therapy. Medication nonadherence is a major risk factor for both nonresponse and relapse. Causes of nonadherence include intolerance of side effects, inadequate psychoeducation, avoidance of dealing with issues of stigma or shame (associated with the illness), and strains in the physician-patient alliance. When the prescriber is also a psychotherapist, it is easy to make time to address these matters. A nonmedical psychotherapist also may be able to facilitate adherence without triangulation (i.e., splitting). Given the brevity and infrequency of medication management visits in most community settings, the collaborating

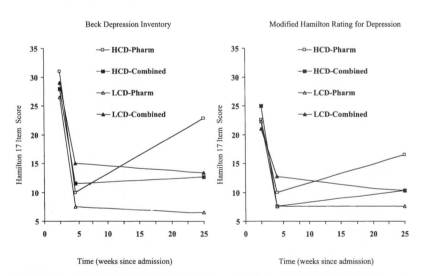

FIGURE 2 Miller, Norman, and Keitner (1990) found that the combination of CBT (cognitive behavioral therapy) and antidepressant medication was particularly effective among patients with high levels of dysfunctional attitudes. (Reprinted, with permission, from Miller, Norman, & Keitner, 1990.)

psychotherapist may contribute by helping to address issues raised by pharmacotherapy (see Section 4).

PRACTICAL ISSUES

There are two ways to provide combination treatments. In a split-treatment model a psychotherapist collaborates with a primary care physician or psychiatrist. With an integrated model a psychiatrist provides both psychotherapy and pharmacology. Both cost and a shortage of psychiatrists necessitate the split-care model. There is however a paucity of evidence regarding the superiority of one approach over the other. Psychiatrists often believe that the integrated model is optimal. One plus in favor of the single provider is the likelihood of clear and nonconflicting psychoeducation about the treatment plan (when compared with a pair of providers). Similarly a single provider precludes the possibility of the splitting of communication (Thase, 1996). Nevertheless, there is little evidence that such splitting commonly disrupts care provided by a psychiatrist-psychotherapist team. It should be recognized that there are substantial guild-based advantages to the single provider model. The occasional problems that arise because of miscommunication between the providers usually can be addressed by telephone or e-mail.

The split treatment model is favored by most managed care organizations because of lower costs. The actual cost of a single provider model is typically overestimated by the managers of healthcare systems, because psychiatrists tend to treat more severely ill patients for longer periods of time (Wells, Burnam, Rogers, Hays, & Camp, 1992). However, after controlling for case complexity, the extra cost of psychiatric care tends to disappear (Dewan, 1999; Goldman, McCulloch, Cuffel, Zarin, Suarez, & Burns, 1998). Randomized studies of integrated or split treatment are needed to resolve the issue of cost effectiveness of each models.

ARE PSYCHIATRISTS EVEN NECESSARY?

There has never been an RCT that compared the pharmacotherapy outcomes of psychiatrists with those of primary care physicians.

Results of one nonrandomized study suggest that pharmacotherapy provided by a psychiatrist was superior (Blackburn et al., 1981). Specifically, antidepressant pharmacotherapy was virtually ineffective in the subset of depressed patients treated by primary care physicians, whereas it was quite effective in the subset of patients treated by psychiatrists. The outcome of the treatment as usual (i.e., antidepressants prescribed by primary care physicians) was also quite poor in several other studies (Teasdale et al., 1984; Schulberg et al., 1996). On the basis of very limited data, we suggest that patients with complex, comorbid disorders, such as an episode of major depression superimposed on long-standing posttraumatic stress disorder or substance abuse, may do best if combined treatment is provided by a psychiatrist (Thase, 1997).

PHARMACOTHERAPY: APPROVAL AND REGULATION

The United States Food and Drug Administration (FDA) requires 3 phases of research before it approves of a new psychotropic medication. Phase I involves the demonstration of safety and an estimation of therapeutic dosage, and principally involves normal, healthy volunteers. The second and third phases are used to establish efficacy in studies using progressively more sophisticated research designs. These studies are conducted double-blind and must use random assignment and parallel groups. The first goal is to establish efficacy in comparison to an inert placebo. Despite ethical concerns about the use of placebo (e.g., Michaels, 2000), the FDA continues to require the completion of at least two positive placebo-controlled studies before granting approval for general use of a psychotropic medication. Thereafter, studies also may include an active comparator drug (i.e., a treatment that has already received FDA approval).

At the time of approval, it is not necessary to determine if a new medication is more effective than already available medications. Thus, most psychotropic medications are approved before there is much data on relative efficacy. The effect sizes of antidepressant and antianxiety medications are only modestly (0.2–0.4) superior to placebo (Khan et al., 2000; Walsh et al., 2002). In fact, FDA-approved medications fail to show a statistically significant drug-placebo difference in approximately 50% of controlled clinical trials of antidepressants and anxiolytics (Thase, 1999). The proportion of failed trials of antimanic and antipsychotic medications has been smaller (on the order of 25–35%), and effect sizes are typically in the moderate range. This is because patients with more severe and disabling disorders have a lower placebo response rate.

Safety data from 1000–2000 patients are available at the time a novel compound is introduced. Most patients with severe medical conditions are excluded from phase 2 and phase 3 clinical trials, however, which limits the knowledge about the safety of novel medications. Post-marketing (phase 4) studies are necessary to gain further information on side effects, toxicities, and tolerability.

Though the FDA approval of a new medication is granted initially for treatment of one specific disorder, many psychotropics have therapeutic effects that extend across diagnostic boundaries. For example, although most antipsychotic medications are approved for treatment of schizophrenia, they are widely prescribed for treatment of mania and psychotic depression. Other current examples of "off-label" use are prescription of the anticonvulsant carbamazepine for the management of mania and the antidepressant trazodone an hypnotic for the treatment of insomnia. Off-label use sometimes precedes eventual FDA approval, as was the case with anticonvulsants divalproex and lamotrigine and the antipsychotic olanzapine as treatments for bipolar disorder. Conversely, off-label use may continue for years (or even decades) without formal approval (e.g., tricyclic antidepressants for treatment of panic disorder). This is often simply a business decision: Seeking FDA approval for a specific indication involves a manufacturer's commitment of up to $40,000,000 for research and development. Thus, costs must be weighed against the prospects for a return on the investment, which depends on factors such as the prevalence of the disorder, drug industry competition, and the number of remaining years of the drug's patent life.

THE GENERAL APPROACH TO PHARMACOTHERAPY

Pharmacotherapeutic management of most mental disorders is palliative, not curative. Psychopharmacologists face the same issues as managing physicians who are treating patients with hypertension, diabetes, and arthritis. The aims of pharmacotherapy are to suppress symptoms, restore premorbid ("normal self") functioning, and prevent relapses or chronicity. Monitoring the frequency and severity of signs and symptoms of patients' specific disorders enables the psychopharmacologist to assess response to pharmacotherapy. Formal rating scales usually are not used to measure outcomes. Instead, most physicians rely on global impressions and patient's reports of benefits.

Pharmacotherapy of most disorders follows three distinct phases: acute, continuation, and maintenance. The acute phase of pharmacotherapy may last anywhere from a few weeks to months if a patient is not responsive to treatment. Frequency of visits may range from weekly to monthly, with the weekly sessions preferred for patients with suicidal ideation or florid symptoms. The acute phase ends when a full remission or a marked global response to treatment is achieved. The goals of the next, or continuation phase, are prevention of relapse and consolidation and generalization of improvements. The visit frequency typically changes to monthly or bimonthly. The focus of medical management shifts to issues of adherence, longer-term side effect concerns (i.e., weight gain or sexual dysfunction), and self-monitoring of signs and symptoms of impending relapse. For disorders with a better prognosis (e.g., a first episode of depression or panic disorder), pharmacotherapy is usually tapered and discontinued after 6–12 months of sustained remission. For more chronic and/or recurrent disorders, the continuation phase is followed by an indefinite course of maintenance-phase therapy.

Maintenance-phase visits are usually infrequent. After months of well-being, patients are seen quarterly, twice yearly, or even annually. Although some consider maintenance-phase therapy to be life-long, there are sufficient grounds for optimism (i.e., development of more curative treatments) that we prefer to use the term "indefinite." Medication dosages should not be lowered unless there are serious problems with side effects.

Pharmacotherapy for most mental disorders follows a disease-management model, although there are differences in the physician's approach to treatment of medical and psychiatric conditions. Foremost, psychiatrists generally view psychopathology from a broader biopsychosocial perspective. Factors such as social support, adversity, and coping styles are taken into account, and the treatment plan is individualized on the basis of a multiaxial case formulation.

People suffering from psychiatric conditions also differ from those with most other medical problems because of the greater potential effects of societal stigma. Some continue to view mental illness as a sign of character weakness. From this vantage point, use of psychotropic medication(s) may be belittled as a crutch or a cop-out. The person with diabetes rarely is taunted about being "hooked" on insulin.

Moreover, the more severe psychiatric disorders affect judgment and the ability to use abstract thought; this can compromise the ability to understand and truly collaborate in treatment decisions. Together, these problems underscore the importance of involving the family as part of the treatment alliance.

Mental health treatment is regrettably still hampered by limited access. There is a lack of parity in insurance benefits between mental health treatment, if covered at all, and general medical care. Adequate low-cost mental health care for the indigent and working poor is seldom available.

DISORDERS THAT MAY RESPOND BETTER TO COMBINED TREATMENT THAN TO PSYCHOTHERAPY ALONE

Controlled studies demonstrate that 40–70% of patients with major depressive disorder (nonpsychotic nonmelancholic subtype), dysthymia, panic disorder, obsessive-compulsive disorder (OCD), social phobia, generalized anxiety disorder (GAD), bulimia, and primary insomnia achieve a satisfactory response with psychotherapy alone (American Psychiatric Association, 1992, 1998; Smith, 2002). These response rates are superior to the spontaneous remission rates observed in waiting-list control groups, and generally surpass the gains observed in pseudotherapy or attentional control conditions. The only caveat is that the evidence derived from RCTs of well-specified therapies may not generalize to the most commonly practiced eclectic psychotherapies. The existence of effective pharmacotherapies for each of these conditions creates options for patients and issues such as preference, availability, and cost must be considered.

Depressive Disorders

Cognitive behavior therapy (CBT) and interpersonal psychotherapy (IPT) have been widely studied in RCTs of combined strategies. No controlled studies of strategy combinations utilizing psychodynamic psychotherapy and pharmacotherapy have yet been published.

Meta-analyses of studies of depressed outpatients have shown relatively small additive effect sizes for CBT and IPT (Conte, Plutchik, Wild, & Karasu, 1986; Depression Guideline Panel, 1993). The modest nature of these additive effects are still important, however, because each monotherapy also would be expected to have only a small advantage relative to placebo. Some patient subgroups may gain even greater benefit. For example, in a pooled analysis of nearly 600 depressed patients (Thase, Greenhouse, et al., 1997), the authors concluded that pharmacotherapy plus IPT resulted in a 15% greater remission rate when compared with either IPT and CBT alone. However, combined treatment produced a much larger additive effect among patients with severe, recurrent depression (Figure 3).

DiMascio and collegues (1979) conducted the single, most influential study of IPT and pharmacotherapy for treatment of major depressive disorder. The clinicians compared IPT and amitriptyline, singly and in combination. A low contact treatment-on-demand condition served as the comparison group. Both monotherapies were superior to the control group and the combination was more effective than the monotherapies on some symptom measures. A later analysis of these data (Prusoff, Weissman, Klerman, & Rounsaville, 1980) revealed that all three active treatment groups were simarly effective for the subset of patients with the situational, nonendogenous subtype major depressive disorder, whereas combined treatment was superior to monotherapies among the patients with nonsituational, endogenous depression (see Thase, 2000, for a further discussion of this interaction). Although this post-hoc analysis could not exclude the possibility of chance variation, the findings exactly parallel those of Thase, Greenhouse, and colleagues (1997). Thus, severe, recurrent (i.e., endogenous) depression can be considered a disorder for which combined treatment would be effective.

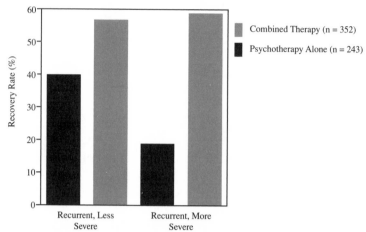

FIGURE 3 Recovery rates in patients in midlife (younger than 60 years) with recurrent major depression as a function of severity and treatment type. (Reprinted, with permission, from Thase, Greenhouse, et al., 1997.)

Most of the first wave of individual studies employing cognitive or behavioral therapies have failed to show a statistically significant additive benefit of a combined treatment approach (Beck, Hollon, Young, Bedrosian, & Budenz, 1985; Hersen et al., 1984; Hollon et al., 1992; Murphy et al., 1984). However, these studies were designed and completed before the concepts of statistical power and design were widely appreciated. None of the trials had adequate statistical power to detect even moderate additive effects (i.e., a 15–20% difference in remission rates). Moreover, results may have been affected by use of tricyclic antidepressants, which may be relatively ineffective in the treatment of younger depressed women (Thase, Frank, Kornstein, & Yonkers, 2000). This is particularly true for depressed patients with reverse neurovegetative features (e.g., overeating or oversleeping) (Quitkin et al., 1993; Stewart, Garfinkel, Nunes, Donovan, & Klein, 1998). Stronger additive results may have been observed if better tolerated medication had been available (see, for example, Keller et al., 2000).

The investigations of two small studies of hospitalized depressed patients found evidence favoring combined strategy over medication management alone (Bowers, 1990; Miller, Norman, & Keitner, 1989). As discussed previously, Miller and collegues (1990) found a large additive effect among the patients with high levels of dysfunctional attitudes. Such patients also tend to respond less favorably to CBT alone (Whisman, 1993). Although the data are sparse, the combination of CBT and pharmacotherapy may be especially useful for depressed patients who require hospitalization.

There have been two published studies of combined treatment of chronic depression. Ravindran and collegues (1999) found little evidence of an additive effect for CBT (conducted as group therapy) and sertraline in a study of 97 outpatients with dysthymia. However, in this study group, CBT was no more effective than placebo. In a multicenter trial of over 650 patients with chronic forms of depression, Keller and collegues (2000) compared an individual therapy specifically developed for management of chronic depression, cognitive behavior analysis system of psychotherapy (CBAS; McCullough, 2000), and pharmacotherapy with nefazodone, alone and together. They found that the group receiving combined treatment had substantially better response and remission rates than both of the monotherapies, which had virtually identical outcomes (Figure 1). Although comparably effective, nefazodone had earlier symptomatic benefits than CBASP, especially on measures of sleep disturbance (Thase et al., 2002).

In an early study of continuation therapy, Klerman, DiMascio, Weissman, Prusoff, and Paykel (1974) found that combined treatment was no more effective than pharmacotherapy alone in preventing relapses. However, this study does not fairly represent the therapeutic potential of IPT, as all of the patients had responded to amitriptyline before they began psychotherapy. Moreover, there was a later-emerging trend that suggested that the patients who had received individual psychotherapy (a forerunner of IPT) and who had not relapsed obtained a significantly higher level of social adjustment.

Two more recent studies have evaluated the efficacy of combined treatment in the maintenance phase of recurrent depression. In both of these studies, patients were treated with IPT and TCAs (tricyclic antidepressants) during the acute and continuation phases. In the first study (Frank et al., 1990), which involved 125 patients between the ages of 19 and 65 and whose symptoms had remitted, continued monthly IPT sessions in combination with high-dose imipramine was no more effective in preventing recurrence than imipramine alone across 3 years of maintenance treatment. Monthly IPT sessions (either alone or with placebo) did provide some prophylaxis when compared to a placebo condition. Further, IPT's preventive effects were significantly stronger when therapist-patient dyads were able to sustain focus on interpersonal problems (Frank et al., 1990; Spanier et al., 1996). In other words, if IPT "devolved" into nonspecific support, it had no demonstrable prophylactic benefit.

In the second study, 107 depressed outpatients age 60 and above participated in the double-blind, placebo-controlled maintenance-phase study (Reynolds et al., 1999). In this study, nortriptyline was used instead of imipramine. The findings differed from the first (Frank et al., 1990) in several respects: combined treatment was superior to nortriptyline alone and IPT and pharmacotherapy alone had comparable effects

Another important line of research regards combining treatments in sequence (i.e., adding psychotherapy or pharmacotherapy to treat residual symptoms in patients who have undergone one therapy alone). Fava, Grandi, Zielezny, Canestrari, and Morphy (1994) demonstrated a significant additive effect when a 3-month course of CBT was added to the treatment of patients who had persistent residual symptoms despite pharmacotherapy. In a follow-up report on this study, the CBT-treated group had a significantly better chance of discontinuing medication without relapse (Fava, Grandi, Zielezny, Rafanelli, & Canestrari, 1996), as well as a sustained decrease in recurrence risk (Fava, Rafanelli, Grandi, Canestrari, & Morphy, 1998). Paykel and colleagues (1999) extended these findings in a multicenter study of incompletely remitted patients. The group that received CBT in addition to continued pharmacotherapy had about a 50% reduction in relapse risk as compared to the group receiving only pharmacotherapy. The protective effect of sequential CBT against recurrent depression was also shown in another study by the Bologna group (Fava, Rafanelli, Grandi, Conti, & Belluardo, 1998). In this small but informative trial, 20 fully remitted patients received either a 14-session course of CBT or supportive medication management prior to withdrawal of antidepressants. CBT significantly reduced the risk of recurrence over the following 2 years.

Thase, Buysse, and collegues (1997) reported on the opposite strategy—adding an antidepressant (either imipramine or fluoxetine) after nonresponse to individual IPT. A 76% remission rate was observed among 38 patients in this case series. Interpretation of this study is limited by the lack of a placebo control. Nevertheless, it is improbable that such a high remission rate would be observed after 2–4 months of unsuccessful psychotherapy due to nonspecific factors alone (see Stewart, Mercier, Agosti, Guardino, & Quitkin, 1993). Frank, Grochocinski, and collegues (2000) subsequently observed similar results in a second group of IPT nonresponders.

Panic Disorder

Effective treatments for panic disorder include several forms of CBT, a number of antidepressants, and potent benzodiazepines. Comparisons between different treatment modalities typically show parity; preference for CBT is based on avoidance of medication side effects and greater durability of gains (American Psychiatric Association, 1998).

Although benzodiazepines are rapidly effective for treatment of panic disorder, liability for abuse, development of tolerance of therapeutic effects, and difficulty of withdrawal are major drawbacks. Sequenced therapy with CBT has been shown to facilitate successful discontinuation of benzodiazepines (Otto et al., 1993; Spiegel et al., 1994).

Studies of combined benzodiazepine and CBT have failed to show any meaningful additive effect (Spiegel & Bruce, 1997). For example, studies using moderate doses of lower potency benzodiazepines such as diazepam did not show additive effects (Hafner & Marks, 1976; Wardle, 1990). There is also the theoretic concern that medication effects might compromise memory and learning during exposure therapy (Curran, 1986). A two-center randomized trial comparing alprazolam (versus placebo) and exposure therapy (versus relaxation) in 154 outpatients with panic disorder and agoraphobia addressed this issue. Results failed to support the value of adding alprazolam (up to 5mg per day) to exposure therapy

(Marks et al., 1993). Furthermore, combination treatment was superior to alprazolam alone.

The only advantages observed in the groups treated with alprazolam were observed in the first four weeks of therapy (Marks et al., 1993). A small early advantage for combined treatment with benzodiazepines and CBT must be weighed against longer-term outcomes. In this study, the relapse rate following discontinuation of alprazolam was approximately 50%, as compared to only 12% for patients who received therapy and placebo (Basoglu, Marks, Swinson et al., 1994). The link between relapse risk and drug withdrawal was mediated by patients' attributions that the medication "caused" their improvement to the benzodiazepine (Basoglu, Marks, Kilic, Brewin, & Swinson, 1994).

Thus, it seems unlikely that benzodiazepines actually disrupt learning *per se*, in therapy. Rather it appears that pharmacotherapy may reduce patients' confidence in the *in vivo* exposure strategies that are crucial in the success of behavioral treatment. Therefore, if a benzodiazepine is prescribed in combination with CBT to try to hasten symptomatic improvement, it would be important to emphasize the potentially enduring value of the psychotherapy and perhaps even to minimize the contribution of pharmacotherapy. Also, when the benzodiazepine is tapered, it should be withdrawn gradually in concert with *in vivo* exposure or CBT strategies.

Most experts now favor antidepressants for combined treatment for panic disorder (American Psychiatric Association, 1998). In the largest such study, Barlow, Gorman, Shear, and Woods (2000) evaluated the outcomes of 312 outpatients with panic disorder. The study followed a 2x2 factorial design: patients were randomized to placebo versus imipramine and to CBT versus clinical management. A fifth cell, CBT alone, was added to determine if placebo adversely affected therapy outcomes. The monotherapies were both significantly more effective than placebo in the intent-to-treat analyses of 3-month outcomes; there was no evidence that placebo diminished the efficacy of CBT. The combination of CBT and imipramine was significantly more effective than pharmacotherapy alone, but no more effective than CBT plus placebo. By the end of the continuation phase, the advantages of combined treatment dissipated after withdrawal of imipramine.

The SSRIs (selective seratonin reuptake inhibitors) have replaced TCAs for first-line treatment of panic disorder. Given their better tolerability, it may be easier to demonstrate an advantage for SSRI + psychotherapy combination in future studies. The SSRIs are also well suited for longer term use.

Unlike benzodiazepines, antidepressants do not rapidly suppress somatic cues of arousal, and therefore do not undercut the value of exposure. Therefore, antidepressants can be used for longer periods of time than benzodiazepines in the treatment of panic disorder. Nevertheless, discontinuation of effective antidepressants is still associated with a risk of relapse, which may again justify the use of sequential treatment strategies.

Obsessive Compulsive Disorder

Behavior therapy and selected antidepressants with strong serotonergic activity are the best-established treatments for OCD. Controlled studies of behavior therapy or pharmacotherapy with either SSRIs or the TCA clomipramine have consistently failed to show better than 60% response rates in OCD. Moreover, some OCD patients are frightened by thoughts about exposure plus response prevention and decline participation (Mavissakalian, 1995). There are, of course, other drawbacks to pharmacotherapy. At the doses of serotonergic antidepressants used to treat OCD, 10–15% of patients experience intolerable side effects (Griest, Jefferson, Kobak, Katzelnick, & Serlin, 1995). A significant minority of patients experience longer-term side effects such as weight gain or sexual dysfunction.

Several studies of ambulatory OCD patients (Marks, Stern, Mawson, Cobb, & McDonald, 1980; Mawson, Marks, & Ramm, 1982; O'Connor, Todorov, Robillard, Borgeat, & Brault, 1999) have shown significant additive effects for combined therapy, although results are not unanimous (van Balkom et al., 1998). There are several large studies underway that should permit a stronger assessment of the magnitude of additive effects. It seems likely that the best evidence of additive effects will come from large studies of patients with more chronic, severe, or relapsing forms of OCD.

Other Anxiety Disorders

Social anxiety disorder, GAD and PTSD can also be effectively treated with either pharmacotherapy or focused forms of psychotherapy.

The best-studied forms of psychotherapies are behavior therapy and CBT. Effective pharmacotherapies include most types of anti-depressants, buspirone (GAD only), benzodiazepine (GAD only) and beta blockers or B-blockers (social anxiety disorder only).

These disorders are not well-studied and there are virtually no pivotal studies examining the effects of combined treatment (Beaudry, 1991; Mavissakalian, 1995). In the largest study published to date 387 patients with social anxiety disorder were randomized to treatment with either sertraline, placebo and either a brief exposure intervention or supportive care. Although the behavioral treatment was ineffective alone, it did enhance outcomes on a number of dependent measures when used in combination with sertraline (Blomhoff et al., 2001). The poorer longitudinal outcomes of patients suffering from GAD and PTSD make it logical to consider combined treatments.

Bulimia Nervosa and Other Eating Disorders

Bulimia nervosa is responsive to a number of different treatments, including IPT (Fairburn et al., 1991), supportive-dynamic therapy (Freeman, Barry, Dunkeld-Turnbull, & Henderson, 1988), and anti-depressant medication (Walsh & Devlin, 1995). Although there are clearly individual differences in treatment responsiveness, results of several head-to-head comparisons have favored CBT over pharmacotherapy (Agras et al., 1992; Mitchell et al., 1990).

There have been 3 published RCTs of combined treatment of bulimia. Mitchell and collegues (1990) conducted the first large, factorial (2x2) study of 171 bulimic outpatients. They found significantly greater improvement on measures of depression and anxiety among patients treated with imipramine and CBT, as compared to patients treated with CBT plus placebo. However, combined treatment group did not result in a greater reduction of binge eating or vomiting. Combined treatment was significantly more effective than pharmacotherapy alone on most outcome measures. Of note, patients in the imipramine alone group received a substantially more vigorous trial of medication (mean 267mg per day vs. 217mg per day).

Walsh and collegues (1997) studied 120 bulimic outpatients in a 16–week, five cell trial. Four treatment cells received one of two types of psychotherapy, CBT or psychodynamic supportive therapy, in combination with either active pharmacotherapy or placebo (in a 2x2 design). The fifth treatment cell received unblinded pharmacotherapy alone. The pharmacotherapy consisted of a two-stage intervention: the noradrenergic TCA desipramine (up to 300mg per day) followed, if necessary by the SSRI fluoxetine (up to 60mg/day). Overall, pharmacotherapy was superior to placebo, and CBT was more effective than supportive-dynamic psychotherapy. There was evidence of an additive effect for the combination of CBT and active pharmacotherapy, although supportive-dynamic therapy did not improve responses to medication.

In the third trial of combined treatment, Agras and collegues (1992) compared CBT and desipramine, alone and together, in a study of 71 bulimic outpatients. The combined approach was more rapidly effective than CBT alone, but few significant differences remained at week 16. Combined treatment was more effective than desipramine alone on most measures throughout the trial. Continued CBT also protected against relapse after desipramine was discontinued. The efficacy of desipramine was undercut by nonadherence. (Although DMI plasma levels normally can be estimated by about 1.0 to 1.2 times the daily dose, in this study a mean dose of 156.7mg per day produced a mean serum level of only 131ng/ml or about 0.8 of the daily dose.)

Together, these studies suggest that CBT, either alone or in combination with pharmacotherapy, is superior to pharmacotherapy alone. Although the data are far from conclusive, it appears that patients do gain greater benefit from combined treatment. Further studies are needed to determine if a subset of patients who benefit from combined treatment can be identified before treatment is initiated. Further research using multistage sequential treatment strategies is needed.

Substance-Abuse Disorders

Methadone maintenance and naltrexone are approved for use in the treatment of opiate dependence. For treatment of alcoholism, naltrexone and disulfiram are approved for suppression of cravings and relapse prevention respectively. There are no pharmacotherapies approved for the treatment of cocaine or marijuana dependence.

Psychotherapies that have received empirical support for treatment of substance-dependent patients include CBT and supportive-dynamic psychotherapy. Woody and collegues (1983) found that both of these therapies improved outcomes in a study of opiate dependent patients receiving concomitant methadone maintenance therapy. This effect was largely delimited to the subgroup of patients with higher levels of anxiety or depressive symptoms (Woody, McLellan, & Luborsky, 1984). In a more recent study, the combination of CBT and tricyclic desipramine had significant additive effects for a subset of cocaine dependent patients, with concomitant depressive symptoms (Carroll et al., 1994). Disulfiram similarly improved outcomes when added to a contingency based behavioral intervention in a study of alcoholism (Higgins et al., 1991).

These studies provide some basis for optimism about further development of cost-effective psychosocial treatments for substance abusers, but "more" is not always better. In a recent study of more than 400 cocaine dependent patients, the addition of CBT or supportive-dynamic therapy to standard group drug counseling did not improve outcome (Crits-Christoph et al., 1999). Providing professional psychotherapy in addition to group drug counseling was actually significantly less effective than adding sessions of individual drug counseling (Crits-Christoph et al., 1999).

COMBINING TREATMENTS: CONDITIONS THAT SHOULD NOT BE TREATED WITH PSYCHOTHERAPY ALONE

Patients with schizophrenia or mania should not be treated with psychotherapy alone (Thase, 2000). This is because specific pharmacotherapy has clear-cut efficacy in these disorders, whereas there is virtually no evidence that psychotherapy alone is effective. To knowingly withhold pharmacotherapy from patients with these disorders is tantamount to malpractice. Indeed, guardianship procedures may be necessary when pharmacotherapy is indicated as a life-saving treatment.

Psychotherapy as an Adjunctive Therapy: Schizophrenia and Related Disorders

The principal adjunctive psychosocial interventions now used with people with schizophrenia include milieu therapy, CBT, behavior therapy aimed at improving social skills, and various types of family intervention. The scope of these interventions has been evaluated at different stages of treatment, including acute hospitalization, immediately following discharge, and during long-term maintenance care.

Effectiveness of adjunctive inpatient psychosocial interventions for schizophrenia has been extensively evaluated (Lauriello, Bustillo, & Keith, 1999). Several early, large inpatient studies did show modest additive effects for insight-oriented psychotherapy in combination with antipsychotic medications (Grinspoon, Ewalt, & Shader, 1972; May, 1968). The extended length of hospitalizations in these studies (months), however, makes the findings of these studies virtually irrelevant to current practice. Other studies conducted during the same era suggested that longer hospital stays did not add to the benefit of briefer hospitalizations (e.g., Caffey, Galbrecht, & Klett, 1971; Herz, Endicott, & Spitzer, 1977). A subsequent meta-analysis of 26 controlled studies revealed a lack of benefit of psychosocial interventions during shorter, acute-care hospitalization (Lauriello, Bustillo, & Keith, 1999).

The trend of deinstitutionalizing patients with schizophrenia throughout the 1960s and 1970s led to greater focus on the impact of outpatient psychosocial interventions. The goals of intervention in this generation of studies were improved medication adherence, reduction in relapse and rehospitalization rates, improved social functioning, and better tolerance of psychosocial stressors. It is important to note that until recently, psychosocial interventions did *not* aim to directly reduce the positive symptoms of schizophrenia (i.e., delusions and hallucinations). Perhaps the most noteworthy modifiable risk factor was recognition that residing with significant others who manifested a high level of expressed emotion greatly increased the risk of psychotic relapse and rehospitalization (Brown, Birley, & Wing, 1972; Butzlaff & Hooley, 1998; Vaughn & Leff, 1976).

A number of outpatient studies of specific psychosocial interventions have been completed. In such studies, supportive individual interventions such as major role training (Schooler et al., 1980), occupational therapy (Liberman, Wallace, Blackwell, Kopelowicz, Vaccaro, & Mintz, 1998), and personal therapy (Hogarty et al., 1997) have yielded modest additive effects. Interestingly, Hogarty and colleagues (1997) found that personal therapy actually increased the risk of relapse for those living alone. The reasons for this unexpected finding remain unclear. One possibility is that some schizophrenic individuals live alone because they have a low threshold for interpersonal interaction. The well-meaning therapist thus may be perceived as intrusive or even a threat. The benefits of personal therapy thus were limited to those who continued to live with families, which may reflect a better ability to maintain significant social relations.

Family-focused treatments have shown consistency in reducing risk of relapse and improving social function (Falloon et al., 1985; Penn & Mueser, 1996; Randolph et al., 1994). In the study by Randolph and colleagues (1994), for example, a 25-session behavior family management program reduced the risk of relapse from 55% to 14%. Curiously, benefit of the family intervention was not limited to the subset of patients with high expressed emotion. One recent study found that family intervention was helpful even when diluted to a low-intensity, once a month group strategy (Schooler et al., 1997).

Social skills training also has received extensive evaluation. Social skills training has been found to be more effective than supportive therapy control conditions on measures of residual symptoms and social adjustment, as well as *in vivo* behavioral tests (Hogarty et al., 1986; Liberman, Wallace, Blackwell, Kopelowicz, Vaccaro, & Mintz, 1998; Marder et al., 1996). In the study by Hogarty and colleagues (1986), an additive effect was evident between individual skills training and psychoeducational family therapy. In a recent report, beneficial effects of social skills training were sustained across a 2-year follow-up (Liberman et al., 1998). Overall, the addition of social skills training to medication management seems to reduce the risk of rehospitalization (Benton & Schroeder, 1990), although results were not consistent across various studies.

A modified version is also receiving increasing attention as an adjunctive treatment for schizophrenia. Therapy is geared toward helping patients learn to recognize, challenge, and modify psychotic cognitions (Perris, 1989). CBT showed considerable promise in two British studies (Drury, Birchwood, Cochrane, & MacMillan, 1996; Kuipers et al., 1997). In both trials, addition of weekly individual sessions of CBT resulted in improved symptomatic outcomes. Moreover, further analysis of the data obtained from one trial revealed that improvement following CBT was associated positively with the strength of delusions prior to treatment. If replicated, this is a very important finding because symptomatic severity typically predicts poorer response across a wide range of interventions for schizophrenia. Replication studies are in progress in both the United Kingdom and the United States.

Most psychosocial interventions have not shown impressive results in the treatment of institutionalized schizophrenic patients (Lauriello et al., 1999). However, a systematic program based on contingency management principles did demonstrate improvement on both symptomatic and functional measures (Paul, Tobias, & Holly, 1972; Paul & Lentz, 1977). Furthermore, patients were able to decrease or even discontinue antipsychotic medication. Greater use of contingency-based interventions thus could reduce exposure to antipsychotic medication among institutionalized patients, and hence lower the risk of tardive dyskinesia, a potentially irreversible and disabling neurological condition. Unfortunately, the labor intensive (and expensive) program developed by Paul and Lentz (1977) does not appear to have many advocates in the modern era.

Rosenheck and collegues (1998) conducted a study of 291 treatment-resistant, institutionalized veterans. They compared 122 patients treated with the novel antipsychotic clozapine to 169 patients treated with conventional antipsychotics. Clozapine-treated patients were more likely to participate in supplemental psychosocial therapies, which in turn was associated with better outcomes on measures of quality of life and symptoms. It would be interesting to see if the results of this study could be replicated using less toxic novel antipsychotics (such as risperidone or olanzapine).

There is enough evidence to conclude that individual and family-focused psychotherapeutic interventions have definite beneficial effects when provided in combination with antipsychotic medications. Recent evidence also suggests that CBT may be a promising option for improving the course of schizophrenia.

Bipolar Disorder

When compared to schizophrenia, far fewer studies of combined treatment of bipolar disorder have been conducted. This is perhaps because the therapeutic benefits of lithium salts were overvalued until the early 1990s, resulting in a sense of therapeutic complacency (Sachs & Thase, 2000). Although not as disabling as schizophrenia, bipolar disorder is now recognized to result in profound morbidity and increased mortality (Angst, Sellaro, & Merikangas, 2000). Moreover, evidence about the pathogenic effects of stressful life events (Johnson & Roberts, 1995), high levels of expressed emotion (Butzlaff & Hooley, 1998), marital discord (Miklowitz, 1998), and low social support (Johnson, Winett, Meyer, Greenhouse, & Miller, 1999) provides a strong case for research on the impact of various modalities of psychosocial interventions. Psychotherapies also can be adapted to improve knowledge of and enhance adherence to pharmacotherapy (Cochran, 1984).

The findings of three large studies of adjunctive psychotherapy have been published recently and additional research is ongoing. In the first such report, Perry, Tarrier, Morriss, McCarthy, and Limb (1999) evaluated a brief (average: seven sessions) individual psychoeducation intervention that focused on information about the disorder and its treatment, as well as identification of early warning signs of impending relapse. When compared to a treatment as usual condition, patients who received psychoeducational therapy had a significant reduction in manic relapses.

The second study (Miklowitz et al., 2000) evaluated a longer-term model of family-focused therapy (FFT). A preliminary study of this method involving nine patients in relation to a historical control group (i.e., 1 relapse or 11% versus 14 relapses among 23 controls or 61%) had yielded promising results. Participants of the larger trial had been recently hospitalized for treatment of an acute episode of mania (n=51), depression (n=15), or a mixed state (n=35) and were assigned randomly to receive pharmacotherapy and either clinical management (n=70) or 21 sessions of FFT (n=31) across a 9-month period. Results confirmed the benefit of FFT over the comparison group across the first year, both in terms of fewer depressive relapses and lower levels of depressive symptoms. Of note, these effects were not mediated by improved medication adherence or reduced levels of expressed emotion. However, both of these "predictors" contributed to outcome independent of treatment assignment. The advantage of FFT was most pronounced among patients who had not fully recovered from the index episode.

The third study examined a modified form of IPT, which was adapted to include lifestyle management strategies intended to help bipolar patients to stabilize social rhythms (interpersonal social rhythms therapy or IPSRT; Frank, Swartz & Kupfer, 2000). This study used a 2x2 sequential design with one half of the patients initially receiving IPSRT for acute-phase management (the remainder received clinical management). During the maintenance phase of the study, one-half of the patients received the same treatment strategy, whereas the remainder were assigned to the alternate strategy. All patients received appropriate pharmacotherapy following expert consensus guidelines (American Psychiatric Association, 1993).

The major findings were: (1) IPSRT did indeed significantly enhance patient's lifestyle regularity (Frank et al., 1997), (2) IPSRT did not improve acute-phase treatment outcomes or speed time to remission (Cole et al., 2002; Hlastala et al., 1997), (3) discontinuation of acute phase IPSRT led to an increase in relapse risk, (4) the addition of maintenance IPSRT did not lower relapse risk (Frank et al., 1999), and (5) patients receiving maintenance IPSRT experienced a significant, later-emerging reduction in depressive symptoms and an increase in "well" or euthymic days (Frank et al., in press).

Individual and group forms of CBT also are receiving increasing attention as an adjunctive treatment for bipolar disorder (e.g., Basco & Rush, 1995; Scott, 1996). Although the results of definitive studies have not yet been published, illustrative case series and pilot studies have suggested antidepressant effects (Zaretsky, Segal, & Gemar, 1999) and lower relapse risk (Fava, Bartolucci, Rafanelli, & Mangelli, 2001; Lam et al., 2000; Palmer, Williams & Adams, 1995).

In aggregate, these studies consistently support the use of focused psychosocial treatment with patients receiving pharmacotherapy for bipolar disorder. Family- and interpersonally-oriented interventions appear to help protect against depression whereas psychoeducation and relapse prevention training may reduce risk of manic relapse.

SUMMARY

There is now compelling evidence that focused psychosocial interventions can improve the outcomes of patients with a number of persistent and severe mental disorders. Combined treatment is best established for: schizophrenia; severe, recurrent, or chronic major depressive disorders; obsessive-compulsive disorder; and (most recently) bipolar disorder. Additive effects also have been observed in bulimia and panic disorder, although the results are less consistent. The benefits of combined treatment are partly disorder-specific (e.g., social skills training for schizophrenia) and partly domain-focused (e.g., reduction of expressed emotion in a household or improved medication adherence). Therapy-specific outcomes have not yet been demonstrated.

There is little evidence that psychotherapy-pharmacotherapy combinations should be considered the standard of care for patients with milder depressive and anxiety disorders (the most prevalent conditions for which people seek treatment). The lack of additive effects may justify use of the monotherapies first, based on availability and patient preference, with the alternate strategy used in sequence or in combination if necessary.

There are several areas that warrant future research. At one extreme, whether there are *any* relative indications for combined treatment provided by a single provider is a very important topic. We hypothesize that patients with severe Axis II pathology would be the most likely to benefit from a single provider. At the other end of the continuum, the data on effectiveness of pharmacotherapy as provided by primary-care physicians as prescribers is worrisome. This is based on low patient satisfaction ratings (Seligman, 1995) and poorer outcomes in clinical trials (e.g., Blackburn et al., 1981; Schulberg et al., 1996; Teasdale et al., 1984). As there are too few psychiatrists to provide all the pharmacotherapy for mental disorders, improving the collaborative care provided by psychotherapist-generalist teams must be a considered to be a public health priority.

A new generation of research is needed to evaluate the dissemination of findings from specialty research clinics to everyday practice settings. Treatments that are beneficial only when provided by hand-picked, highly skilled expert therapists offer little value to patients who receive their care in busy urban clinics or community mental health centers.

The Challenges of Split Treatment*

Michelle B. Riba, M.D.

Richard Balon, M.D.

Clinical Case

Charlie, a 52-year-old divorced man with a history of panic disorder and intermittent alcohol abuse, was brought in to the emergency department after neighbors noted that he was not caring for himself. Charlie was morose after a long-term relationship had ended. He said that he had been in therapy with a social worker but had stopped the sessions about 6 months ago due to financial constraints. Charlie noted that he received an antidepressant medication from a psychiatrist whom he saw every 3 months but had missed his last appointment. Both the social worker and psychiatrist were called by the emergency staff. The social worker did not carry a beeper and her voicemail said she was away for 2 weeks. The psychiatrist was unaware that Charlie had stopped his psychotherapy appointments and had lost track of the patient after the missed appointment.

This case example represents split therapy at its worst: poor communication between clinicians, a patient who gets lost to fol-

* Reprinted with permission from Kay, J. (Ed.), Integrated treatment of psychiatric disorders (Review of Psychiatry Series, Volume 20, Number (Oldham, J. M. and Riba, M. B., series editors). Washington, DC: American Psychiatric Publishing.

low-up, a social worker who does not maintain coverage when away—altogether, a system of care that doesn't provide maximum benefit for the patient. Although not all split treatment is bad, there are areas of concern that merit in-depth discussion. This chapter examines the positive and negative aspects of split treatment and presents some clinically useful ways to optimize this type of care.

OVERVIEW

The term *split treatment* is not universally accepted; the literature employs various terms (Table 1) to denote the practice by which a psychiatrist or other physician provides the psychotropic medications while a nonphysician (e.g., social worker, psychologist, counselor) provides the psychotherapy. We will use the term *split treatment* to denote this type of care.

The last time psychiatric guidelines were organized and published on this practice was in 1980, when the American Psychiatric Association drafted a "living document to be adapted to local custom and practice" (American Psychiatric Association, 1980). This publication attempted to review the roles and responsibilities of psychiatrists in the range of consultative, supervisory, and collaborative relationships with other professionals and nonprofessionals

---

TABLE 1

Terms Used as Synonyms for Split Treatment

- Collaborative treatment
- Combined treatment
- Concurrent care
- Divided treatment
- Integrated care
- Med backup
- Medical backup
- Medication check
- Medication management
- Parallel treatment
- Shared treatment
- Triangular (or triangulated) treatment

in a wide variety of systems of care. Since that time, no other set of official psychiatric guidelines has been provided on this subject.

An interesting historical aspect is that early split treatment was generally provided by two physicians, a psychiatrist-prescriber and a psychoanalyst-therapist (Fromm-Reichmann, 1947). The subsequent growth of split treatment has been due to a number of factors, including the increased penetration of nonphysician therapists into mental health services (Beitman, 1983; Goldberg, Riba, & Tasman, 1991; Pilette, 1988) and the expanding role of primary-care physicians (PCPs) in treating the majority of patients with emotional problems in the United States (Horgan, 1985; Regier, Goldberg, & Taube, 1978; Valenstein, 1999). The education and training of nonphysician therapists can vary greatly, as can the psychological bent of PCPs, making split treatment relationships between clinicians highly subjective and individual (Neal & Calarco, 1999).

The explosion of safer and cheaper psychotropic medications (e.g., antidepressants, antipsychotics, anxiolytics, mood stabilizers) has made PCPs and other physicians more comfortable prescribing medications and therefore participating in split treatment. In general, the public has become more educated about the use and value of psychotropic medications. Books such as the best-seller *Listening to Prozac* by psychiatrist Peter Kramer (1992) have made *antidepressant* a household term. There is widespread advertising of psychotropic medication in the print and media. The Internet has allowed consumers to read about and understand medications, and for many has destigmatized mental illness and the psychotropic medications used for its treatment. Patients are no longer surprised when psychotropic medications are offered as part of the treatment plan; in fact, many have come to expect it.

Cost containment and the emphasis of managed care on multidisciplinary care delivery, especially in the outpatient setting, have also contributed to the increased practice of split therapy. Use of less costly nonmedical therapists rather than more expensive psychiatrists to provide psychotherapy to patients has certainly been a strong driving force in recent years (Kerber, 1999). The ensuing role changes for psychiatrists have included moving from treater or provider toward evaluator or consultant. Interestingly, recent studies have asked whether split treatment is indeed more cost-effective and clinically efficient than having a single psychiatrist provide both psychopharmacology and psychotherapy (Goldman, et al., 1998).

Finally, the growing trend toward a decreased emphasis on psychotherapy training in psychiatric resident training may be related to the burgeoning of split treatment (Riba, Goldberg, & Tasman, 1993). A recent article by Mischoulon and colleagues (2000) delineated issues regarding transfer of care of "psychopharmacology patients" from one resident to the next, noting that there has been a shift away from thinking about dynamic issues in such transitions. Residents increasingly are viewing themselves as prescribers of medication rather than as physicians who need to work through the underpinnings of mental illness with their patients (Spitz, Hansen-Grant, & Riba, 1999). The following case reveals such an issue.

Clinical Case

Tracy, a 28-year-old single mother diagnosed with major depression (recurrent with psychotic features) and borderline personality disorder, had been in psychotherapy with a social worker at the community mental health center for 3 years. Tracy had been taking both antidepressants and antipsychotic agents and was recently hospitalized after a serious suicide attempt by overdose. An inpatient conference was held to determine whether Tracy's suicide attempt could have been avoided. The outpatient resident at the community health center was asked to present Tracy's case and proceeded to discuss what medications she had been on and her medical history. When asked about recent psychosocial stressors that could have led to the suicide attempt, he said, "Please ask the social worker. I am Tracy's psychopharmacologist."

The role of the psychiatry resident—in fact, of all psychiatrists—has become increasingly blurred. The provision of psychotherapy, previously viewed as a necessary skill in the armamentarium of psychiatrists and in the training of residents, has ceased to be essential because of the rise of split treatment. In recognition of these problems, the American Psychiatric Association developed its Commission on Psychotherapy by Psychiatrists, and the Residency Review Committee in Psychiatry of the American Medical Association has promulgated new regulations for training in psychotherapy (effective January 2001). Although these actions will help, the fundamental problems regarding split treatment and the identity of psychiatrists with regard to psychotherapy remain.

This discussion of split treatment is meant to provide the reader with a broad sense of the complexity of the issues surrounding this type of care. There are many varieties of professional involved with this system of care; further, split therapy is pervasive in all treatment settings—inpatient, outpatient, community mental health centers, private and managed practices, partial programs, and even emergency settings. The following sections will elaborate on the specific positive and negative aspects of split treatment.

POSITIVE ASPECTS OF SPLIT TREATMENT

When it is practiced well, there are many positive aspects to split treatment (Balon, 1999).

Patients Have More Time with Clinicians

In split treatment, patients have the opportunity to work with at least two clinicians: one nonmedical therapist for psychotherapy and one physician for psychotropic medications. In this arrangement, patients are generally seen by the therapist for 50-minute sessions and by the psychiatrist for 20- to 30-minute sessions. How frequently these sessions occur is dictated by clinical need, fiscal resources and medical benefits, and clinician availability.

Clinicians' vacations may be easier for patients to negotiate in split treatment. For example, if vacations can be planned and staggered, it is helpful for patients to be able to see one clinician when the other is away. This might avoid crises for patients who feel abandoned or angry during clinicians' vacations, as exemplified by the following case.

Clinical Case

Susan, a 19-year-old college sophomore with anorexia nervosa, was doing summer schoolwork when her pregnant therapist delivered her baby 6 weeks earlier than expected. Arrangements were quickly made for Susan's psychiatrist to see the patient more often and to help deal with her therapist's abrupt departure. Susan had very mixed and conflicted emotions during the period of the therapist's absence. The psychiatrist was able to help Susan negotiate many of the wide-ranging mood states and conflicts that arose during this time. When the therapist returned, a session was held with the patient and both clinicians to help with the transition back to Susan's seeing the therapist for psychotherapy.

Because of the greater amount of time spent with clinicians in split therapy, patients may be able to provide more clinically useful information than would be possible with just one clinician. There may be information that the patient feels comfortable sharing with one of the clinicians but not with the other, such as medical issues with the physician. The psychiatrist and therapist should make sure to share such information in order to give the best care possible to the patient (Pilette, 1988).

Better Use of Available Resources

Cost-effective use of resources is important for both patients and clinicians. As there is an increased understanding on the part of PCPs and patients regarding the symptoms of mental illness, there are more patients who recognize the need for quality mental health care. This is good, but the system of care must be expandable enough to provide for those who need it. A multidisciplinary combination of care sources optimally allows for a triage system wherein therapists see patients for mild to moderate symptomatology and more severe cases are referred to psychiatrists. Split treatment lends itself very nicely to this type of triage system because all patients who need psychotropic medication have the benefit of seeing both therapists and physicians. This is illustrated in the following case.

Clinical Case

Cliff, a self-employed construction worker, was hospitalized for an acute myocardial infarction. He was seen by a psychiatrist in the hospital for mild depressive symptoms and felt relieved and helped by this intervention, which included a prescription for an antidepressant. Upon discharge, Cliff was referred to a social worker who was part of his health maintenance organization but was also approved to follow up with the hospital psychiatrist every 2 months.

Greater Choice of Clinicians

Split treatment offers the patient a greater opportunity to choose a clinician who resembles the patient in generation, race or ethnicity, religion, or cultural values. Such matching may help avoid some of the difficulties that arise in psychotherapy when clinician and patient belong to different racial and ethnic groups (Foulks & Pena, 1995). Additionally, such matching could help enhance the therapeutic alliance for patients who might feel uncomfortable with or mistrustful of clinicians of certain backgrounds. Cultural and language barriers have deterred some patients from seeking mental health treatment (Ruiz, Venegas-Samuels, & Alarcon, 1995). Each culture has unique traditions and values that may be misunderstood or misinterpreted by clinicians (Yamamoto, Silva, & Justice, 1993). There has been a greater emphasis in psychiatry residency training on raising such cultural issues and providing better teaching and training. There will, however, always be a gap between what some clinicians know about the values of various cultures and the relative importance of those values in determining patients' psychological problems and psychosocial stressors. As noted by Balon (1999), such factors may play a critical role in the development and presentation of mental illness and in psychotherapy.

Clinical Case

Megumi was a 26-year-old pregnant Japanese woman who accompanied her husband to the United States so that he could study computer engineering. She became quite despondent in the last trimester of her pregnancy and was not eating or sleeping. Members of her church tried to provide support and reassurance. Megumi's shame and guilt over her depression and low self-esteem seemed overwhelming. Her family was quite concerned but refused the obstetrician-gynecologist's referral to a psychiatrist. It was not felt to be culturally appropriate to see a therapist and discuss family problems with someone outside the family system. A social worker of Japanese heritage was found in the community, and the patient agreed to be seen for a consultation.

Another advantage of having two clinicians is the opportunity to capitalize on the unique talents and skills of both. For a 17-year-old anorexic patient who becomes depressed when her parents divorce, it might be optimal to see both a social worker with a specialty in eating disorders and a child and adolescent psychiatrist whose specialty is in the psychopharmacology of mood disorders. In rural areas where there are not enough psychiatrists for the population, it might be especially helpful to balance the psychiatrist's skills with those of a therapist.

Enhanced Professional Support for Clinicians

When split treatment works well, clinicians enjoy a feeling of enhanced collegial support for one another. Split treatment allows for a feeling of mutual caring and for sharing of information that helps clinicians to help each other and the patient through crises. Pilette (1988) noted that this was especially true with difficult patients during difficult times. Patients with borderline personality disorder, for example, are notorious for fueling strong counter-transferential feelings of anger, fear, and worry in clinicians (Silk, 1999). It is therefore quite helpful for clinicians to work together to present the unified message that they can handle the various affective storms presented by certain patients. At the same time, the clinicians can provide a way for each other to diminish burnout with such patients. By sharing the patient and his or her affective storms, split treatment spreads the wealth; the patient with borderline personality disorder has two clinicians to idealize or devalue. When clinicians can recognize and communicate about this with each other and the patient, it may help to clarify and sometimes even calm the situation.

The idea of split therapy enhancing clinicians' emotional support of one another is especially true in a clinic or community health setting where clinicians see each other often and have time to communicate. Psychiatry residents, in particular, value the teaching and support they get from seasoned, mature social workers and psychologists while providing split treatment (Balon, 1999).

In split treatment the therapist has the opportunity to learn more about psychopharmacology and the specific actions and side effects of medications. The physician, with the help of the therapist, has an opportunity to better understand psychodynamic principles. Patients' diagnostic differentials can be discussed between the clinicians, and aspects of personality or medical issues can be deliberated. Psychodynamic principles, transferences, resistances, and defenses are likely to be viewed differently by each clinician. Nevertheless, these differences, if communicated and discussed in a thoughtful manner, can be used in a positive way to better understand and help the patient.

Enhanced Adherence to the Treatment Plan

Patients often strongly resist taking their medication as prescribed. Psychotherapy may either help or hinder medication adherence (Paykel, 1995). In split treatment, the therapist can encourage the patient to stay on the medication while the psychiatrist supports the psychotherapy efforts of the therapist. The patient can ask questions and is educated by both clinicians. Each clinician can advocate for the patient and perhaps help and support the patient through difficult stages of both medication adherence and psychotherapy.

The meaning and role of medication and psychotherapy are critically important. Sometimes patients have difficulty knowing which treatment to value when they are getting better. This is exemplified in the following case.

Clinical Case

Steve, a 56-year-old married man, became quite depressed after being laid off from the job he had held for 22 years. He was in counseling with a social worker, who recommended he be evaluated by a psychiatrist for antidepressant and sleep medication. Within 3 weeks of starting the medications, Steve had decreased vegetative symptoms of depression and felt more like his "old self." He told the psychiatrist that he was planning on stopping therapy with the social worker. The psychiatrist strongly urged Steve to continue in therapy, explaining that the combination of medication and psychotherapy would, in his case, be most helpful. The psychiatrist spoke with the social worker about this and the social worker also conveyed the importance of care by both professionals.

NEGATIVE ASPECTS OF SPLIT TREATMENT

There are also quite a few negative aspects of split treatment (Goldsmith, Paris, & Riba, 1999). Effective split treatment depends upon excellent communication between the patient and clinicians, mutual respect and regard for clinicians' practices, and well-thought-out treatment plans. Often these factors are missing or compromised.

Interdisciplinary Issues

When clinicians know each other and can refer patients to one another for split therapy, they are more comfortable with this system of care (Goldberg, Riba, & Tasman, 1991; Weiner & Riba, 1997). Many times, however, the clinicians in split treatment don't know each other at all. Fueling this unfamiliarity are basic structures in medicine that place physicians at the top and add to feelings of inequality and competition between clinicians (Baggs & Schmitt, 1988). This inequality is sometimes displaced onto the patient during the making of treatment decisions. For example, in fact, some patients are sensitive to this problem and unconsciously exploit the competition between clinicians (Kelly, 1992). Further, there has recently been increased political tension between psychiatrists and psychologists over the issue of prescribing privileges. Finally, the psychotherapy skills and psychopharmacologic education of social workers and psychologists are highly variable (Neal & Calarco, 1999).

It is therefore little wonder that clinicians who don't know each other and who are engaged in split treatment might be wary of one another's strengths and weaknesses. In such circumstances the patient may gain little from the split treatment.

Communication

It is difficult enough for clinicians to keep up with the usual load of paperwork, telephone calls, e-mails, and so on. Yet a major responsibility in split treatment is to communicate with one another. Unfortunately, this is rarely done well (Hansen-Grant & Riba, 1995), and can lead to misperceptions and misunderstanding between clinicians and patients. Even though patients in split treatment should sign explicit consents allowing conversation to occur between clinicians (Appelbaum, 1991), what the limits of such conversations should be and what details may be communicated are often unclear.

Communication issues lead to problems such as not transmitting important information regarding dangerous patient situations, not knowing when the other clinician is going on vacation and assuming that someone will be in town to take care of the patient, making the patient feel that she or he is a messenger between clinicians, misunderstanding or misinterpreting psychodynamic issues as medication side effects, devaluing either psychotherapy or medication indirectly or directly, not having a well-constructed treatment plan, and so on.

Transference and Countertransference

Busch and Gould (1993) have described some of the negative transference reactions that patients may have when their therapists refer them for medication. Such reactions include feeling that the therapist has given up, rejected the patient, or lost interest; overvaluation of the medication and the "chemical imbalance" that supposedly drives the need for medication; idealization of the physician; devaluation of psychotherapy and the therapist; loss of confidence in the therapist; resistance to the exploration of painful issues in psychotherapy; and narcissistic injury and assault on the autonomy of the patient. Busch and Gould note the potential countertransferential feelings of the therapist (shame that he or she was not able to manage the patient completely and needed to ask for help) and that the therapist may be acting out the transference through the referral for medication. Similarly, the countertransferential feelings of the psychiatrist may manifest in colluding with the patient's negative transference toward the therapist and the psychotherapeutic process.

The impact of such negative transference reactions includes the premature closure of the therapeutic process by the patient and a focus on medication to the exclusion of other types of therapy (Bradley, 1990). The physician may unconsciously enjoy being idealized by the patient and the therapist and prescribe medications either too quickly or for too long a period of time, not appreciating the dangers of overreliance on biological interventions. When medication is added to the dyadic relationship between therapist and patient, a four-way relationship is created (Figure 1). Distortions can arise among all four components, leading to unsuccessful treatment and care.

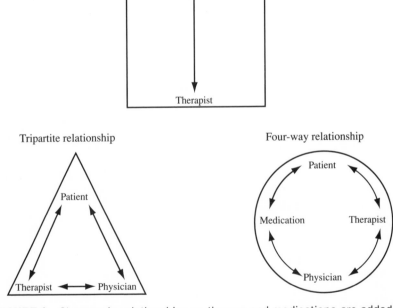

FIGURE 1 Changes in relationships as therapy and medications are added or deleted.

Legal Risks

Another significant problem is the enormous legal risk for psychiatrists who practice split treatment (MacBeth, 1999). Given that the practice of split treatment is now almost ubiquitous, the associated legal issues are all the more troubling for the profession.

What are the sources of liability? In general, there is major potential liability for all psychiatrists who prescribe psychotropic drugs for their patients. Many problems relate to side effects of medication and whether appropriate informed consent is obtained by the physician. Patient suicide or attempted suicide is another significant source of potential liability for psychiatrists who prescribe medication.

Split treatment often heightens or magnifies such problems because patients are essentially shared, leaving the door open for miscommunication between clinicians, missing data, and decreased quality of the doctor-patient relationship. Additionally, information can be misdiagnosed and misunderstood by the patient or clinicians as psychodynamic or physical or both. Valuable time may be lost because of such misunderstandings and therefore lead to legal repercussions. For example, a patient who has recently started taking an antidepressant develops a headache. This can be viewed as resistance (psychodynamic) as a legitimate side effect (physical), or as a combination of both. Patients in split treatment are usually seen less often by the psychiatrist than are patients being seen by the psychiatrist for both psychotherapy and pharmacotherapy. This means psychiatrists don't get to establish the kind of doctor-patient relationship that they would if they were seeing the patient for both psychotherapy and pharmacotherapy (Riba & Tasman, 2000). Similarly, the patient's family might not be as well-known to the psychiatrist. Unfortunately, this area of litigation is burgeoning. (For an in-depth review of this subject, see MacBeth, 1999.)

Ethical Challenges

Although a variety of economic, manpower, and clinical pressures have driven the growth of split treatment, there has been a startling lack of professional oversight or planning for this type of care (Lazarus, 1999). Further, little research has been done on the efficacy or efficiency of split treatment for certain types of patients (Goldman et al., 1998).

Some researchers, in fact, have suggested that managed care not be allowed to dictate split treatment to patients with borderline personality disorder (BPD) because of the inherent intrapsychic splitting defense that already exists in these patients. Patients with personality disorders, especially cluster B diagnoses (American Psychiatric Association, 1994), have disordered interpersonal relationships that often manifest themselves in treatment relationships (Silk, 1999). Such patients often do not tell the same story to both their clinicians (Main, 1957), patients may externalize their problems (Silk, Lee, & Hill, 1995), threaten self-harm (Leibenluft, Gardner, & Cowdrey, 1987), and have substance abuse and emotional lability problems (Springer, Huth, Lohr, & Silk, 1995). Such factors make treatment by two clinicians difficult. As Smith (1989) has written, "in contemporary treatment situations that include a patient, a therapist, a pharmacotherapist, and a pill, the transference issues can become more complex than the landing patterns of airplanes at an overcrowded airport" (p. 80).

When split treatment is the care of choice for a patient, there is, of course, no ethical dilemma. However, if cost considerations become the paramount reason for split treatment, ethical concerns arise.

As Lazarus (1999) has noted there are a variety of potential conflicts when psychiatrists and nonpsychiatrists enter into split treatment relationships. These include conflicts with or around the following:

- State licensing laws.
- Competency questions.
- Physicians being used as figureheads (having authority but not really engaged in the traditional doctor-patient relationship).
- Delegation of medical judgment (by psychiatrists to nonphysician therapists).
- Financial arrangements.

The American Medical Association (1999) and American Psychiatric Association (1997a) have addressed some of the important issues that arise when physicians collaborate with other health and mental health professionals. Still, psychiatrists are often not clear whether they are in a supervisory, consultative, or collaborative relationship with the nonmedical therapist (American Psychiatric Association, 1980), which leads to ethical dilemmas in one of the five categories just listed. Patients, too, are often not clear about how the split treatment is organized and whether or not they have options regarding such care. Further, there is often little discussion between the clinicians and the patient about what would constitute optimal care, because the type of care (i.e., split versus the psychiatrist providing both the therapy and psychopharmacology) is dictated by health care benefits, the training and background of the clinicians (e.g., whether or not the psychiatrist is well-trained to provide psychotherapy), and who sees the patient first.

Clinical Case

Jeff was in psychotherapy with a psychologist for 8 months when he started having rapid cycling of mood swings. A referral was made to a psychiatrist for evaluation and medication management. The patient continued to see both clinicians but the clinicians never spoke with one another. When the psychologist was brought up on the charge of seeing patients without a license, the patient filed an ethics complaint against the psychiatrist with the local American Psychiatric Association district branch, asserting that if the psychiatrist had maintained adequate collaboration with the psychologist, she might have been alerted to the possibility that the psychologist was delivering incompetent care.

Clinical Case

Dr. Brown, a very busy psychiatrist, worked in an office with three social workers and two psychologists. Over a 10-year period Dr. Brown became very comfortable with hearing about his patients from his colleagues and accepting their diagnoses without doing thorough mental status examinations of the patients himself. John, a new patient, was seen by one of the social workers and given the diagnosis of adjustment disorder with depressed mood. Dr. Brown was asked to see the patient in split treatment for medication management. When Dr. Brown saw John, he came into the room saying, "I understand you have some adjustment problems," Dr. Brown saw the patient for less than 10 minutes, did not take a good medical or psychiatric history, and prescribed an antidepressant. Soon thereafter, John was hospitalized on an emergency basis for an insulinoma. The psychiatrist was accused of delegating inappropriate authority to a nonmedical professional.

TOWARD SUCCESSFUL SPLIT TREATMENT

A key aspect of split treatment is how complex and difficult such treatment is for the clinicians, the patient, and the patient's family. Unless the clinician works in a clinic or organized setting where relationships between clinicians are well-delineated (e.g., one psychiatrist works with a specific group of nonmedical therapists), much thought must go into managing safe and effective split treatment.

It may be helpful to think of split therapy having a beginning, middle, and end. In order to avoid or minimize the pitfalls associated with split treatment, the following clinical suggestions are provided as organizing principles for the three stages (Tasman & Riba, 2000):

Beginning of Treatment

- *Communication* is key to providing excellent care in split treatment. At the beginning, both clinicians should obtain a signed release-of-information form from the patient. Communication must be regular and frequent between the clinicians and the patient should be made aware of these discussions. The forms of regular communication should be decided at the outset— routine telephone calls, faxes, e-mails, follow-up letters, and the like. The patient should not be a messenger between the clinicians.
- Issues of *confidentiality* should be discussed at the beginning of treatment. Confidentiality should not be used as a cover to hide from taking the time to make telephone calls, to send copies of evaluations and fol-

low-up notes, to send e-mails or faxes, or to have joint sessions with both clinicians and the patient.

- *Diagnostic impressions* should be independently arrived at, then discussed and agreed upon. If there is a difference of opinion, an understanding must be reached before treatment proceeds.
- The clinicians must work with each other and with the patient to determine the *treatment plan.* The treatment plan should specify how often each of the clinicians expects to see the patient and what process to pursue if the patient doesn't follow up or if there is a missed appointment. If the patient wishes to end the therapy, the medications, or both, it has to be understood that all parties will discuss this important decision.
- It is desirable for a *written contract* to be drawn up between the clinicians and the patient so that all parties understand what the agreement for services will entail. Included in the contract should be a delineation of the clinicians' roles and responsibilities as well as those of the patient.
- Clinicians' *vacation schedules and other on-call and coverage issues* must be discussed regularly and documented. The patient needs to know whom to call in an emergency.
- At the beginning of split treatment, both clinicians and the patient should be aware of their respective *beliefs* regarding medication and psychotherapy.
- There must be a discussion about *what type of care would be optimal for the patient and if there are barriers to such care.* The patient should be informed of this review; if possible, he or she should participate in it.
- The clinician should discuss their *professional backgrounds and training* with each other at the beginning of the patient's treatment. Issues such as licensure, ethics violations, malpractice claims, hospital privileges, coverage of professional liability insurance, participation on managed care panels, and commitment to split treatment should all be made clear.
- The clinicians need to agree *who will communicate with third parties* regarding the patient's care. Further,

each clinician should know the patient's mental health benefits and means of payment. There needs to be an agreement by all parties as to the use of such benefits.

- The clinicians need to understand how best to interface with the patient's *family or significant others.*
- If the patient has health providers other than the psychiatrist and therapist (e.g., primary-care physician, cardiologist, physical therapist), it should be decided which clinician will be the *designated communicator or coordinator* with those other providers.
- At the beginning of treatment there should be a review of how each clinician will assess and manage the patient's thoughts regarding or attempts at *suicide, homicide, violence, and domestic abuse.*
- It should be made clear to the patient what symptoms or types of issues should be brought to the attention of which clinician.
- It is helpful for the clinicians to decide how *problems* will be handled as the need arises.
- The clinicians should discuss differences in fee schedules, cancellation policies, length of visits, and frequency of visits.

Middle Course

- Special attention must be paid to *transference and countertransference* in this system of care. Disparaging and negative remarks made by the patient concerning either clinician, therapy, or medication must be understood and managed in the context of this complex type of treatment.
- Clinicians should review *how many cases of split treatment* they have in their practices and whether or not this is a safe mix. Factors to consider include the clinical complexity of the cases, how busy the practice is, the influence of third-party payers and the hassle factor, the number of different clinicians being worked with, the psychiatric disorders of the patients, and so on. It may be prudent to determine the risks involved in having a large patient population in split treatment

and to weed the number of such patients down to an acceptable level. Further, clinicians should minimize the number of collaborators, since it is virtually impossible to keep track of a large number of clinicians' credentials, vacation schedules, communication patterns, and so on.

- *Adherence to medications and to psychotherapy* should be addressed equally.
- *Treatment plans* should be regularly reviewed and updated between the clinicians and the patient.
- Use of the patient's *mental health benefits* should be regularly reviewed and discussed between clinicians and the patient when appropriate.
- There must be an *agreement that either clinician can terminate the split therapy* but that the patient must be provided adequate and appropriate warning and referrals to other clinicians. In other words, the patient cannot be abandoned.

Ending of Treatment

- After reviewing the treatment plan, both clinicians and the patient should decide together on the *goals* that have been met or not met and the *best time for termination.* They should decide how to stagger the discontinuation of therapy and of medication.
- It is important to consider how to manage *follow-up* and *recurrence of symptoms.*

The clinicians must have a system for giving each other feedback on the care each is providing to the patient. Ideally, after the treatment is complete, the clinicians should review any aspects of the case that could have been managed or handled differently. If possible, the patient should be part of this evaluation process as a way of assuring continuous quality improvement. Most importantly, throughout all stages of the split treatment process, clinicians need to respect both the patient and each other's professional understanding.

Although the challenges of split treatment are great, there are many reasons for clinicians and patients to try to surmount the obstacles. Good communication patterns between clinicians and many of the suggestions noted here can serve as guideposts on the path toward successful split treatment.

Psychodynamic Neurobiology

Barton J. Blinder M.D., Ph.D.

A BIOLOGICAL BASIS FOR MENTAL PROCESSES

In his recent synthesis of his neuroscientific research, LeDoux stated clearly that nature and nurture speak the same language: ". . . they both ultimately achieve their mental and behavioral effects by shaping the synaptic organization of the brain. The particular problem of synaptic connections in an individual's brain and the information encoded by these connections are the keys to who that person is" (2002, p. 3).

Psychotherapy ("psychological therapy") in its varied paradigms and delivery models consists of information exchange, dialogue, and interventions directed toward eliciting change. Achieving psychotherapeutic goals (e.g., insight, affect modulation, decreased relational conflict) depends on some degree of modification to the perceptual, memory, and emotional systems that work both ambiently and enduringly in the brain.

Kandel (1999a) noted that psychoanalysis is "in the best sense a part of biology; it is part of the analysis of mental processes, and these functions must have their foundation in the physical brain. . . there must be a biological basis for the dynamic unconscious, for psychic determinism, for the role of unconscious mental processes in psychopathology, for drives, for transference, and other attachments."

A major focus of psychodynamic psychotherapy is understanding how mental conflict arises from problematic emotional and relational experiences. Individual experiences, with all their complexity and diversity, contribute to and form the autobiographical structure of personality development.

Our concept of *psychoneurosis* (or persisting mental conflict) relates to the encoding of developmental conflictual experiences in representational schemata that are repetitively evoked, leading to nonadaptive, nonerror-correcting responses to the demands of the self-system, relationships, and the material world.

The major dimensions of interest are developmental, psychodynamic, and adaptational. Past experience and habitual modes of reacting and relating magnify and color current mental conflict. In psychotherapy, this leads to psychological defense, resistance, salient dreams, enactment, and transference.

Recent advances in our understanding of brain function associated with cognition, affect, and memory have led to new insight into the impact of experience in the individual processing of memory, emotions, motivation, and dreams (Davis, Charney, Coyle, & Nemeroff, 2002; Geschwind, 2000; Joseph, 1996; LeDoux, 2002; Morisha, 2001; Pally, 1997a, 1997b, 1998a, 1998b).

Selected review of recent research will be discussed to illustrate our expanding knowledge of the neurobiologic bases that contribute to the complex self-system and its potential for conflict. These central problems are the object and focus of psychotherapy.

MEMORY PROCESSING AND THE HIPPOCAMPUS: A DYNAMIC INTERACTION

Memory is the neural representation of information. Its regulation is now understood as having complex temporal and system determinants at significant loci in the brain (Fortin, Agster, & Eichenbaum, 2002; Grigsby & Stevens, 2002; Pally, 1997b; Wall & Messier, 2001). *Iconic* (seconds), *working* (minutes), and *long-term* memory define the operational mnemonic structure. (See Figure 1.) The ability to respond to stimuli and juggle numerous possibilities enables working memory (associated with the frontal lobes—e.g., the dorsolateral prefrontal cortex) to reason rapidly, solve simple problems, and correct errors (Nadel & Moskowitz, 1997; Pally, 1997b; Wicheloren, 1997).

Long-term memory is divided into implicit (outside of awareness) and explicit (declarative, in awareness) memory and has its operational base in the hippocampus with connections to cortex, thalamus, and other sites in the limbic system. The hippocampus serves an index pointing function to other cortical memory sites where memories are consolidated. Explicit memory is further divided into semantic (facts, knowledge) and episodic (spatial, temporal, sensory) memory (Varga-Kahdovan, 1997). The latter may be particularly significant for autobiographical events. Although structures in the medial temporal lobe appear to be necessary for the establishment of long-term memory, they may also be involved in a further consolidation of information through

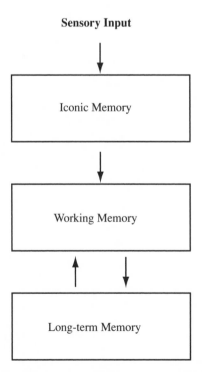

FIGURE 1 Memory sequence showing how brain systems link past, present, and future (Pally, R. (1997b).

higher-order associational cortices—perhaps through active feed-back projections from parahippocampal areas. A significant amount of integration may take place at the hippocampus itself (Lavenex & Amaral, 2000).

Evidence is emerging that the hippocampal formation may also have a role in the attentional control of behavior. The hip-pocampal-orbitomedial prefrontal cortex circuit may be involved in the attentional monitoring of the internal sensorium—a type of working memory of viscero-emotional processing. (See Figure 2.) The hippocampal formation can be viewed as a *discrepancy detec-*

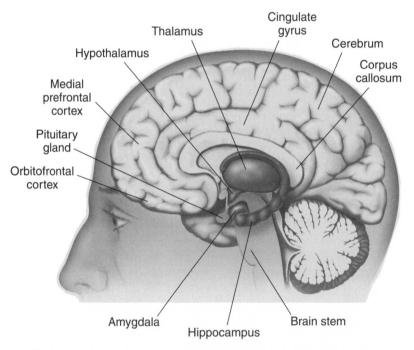

FIGURE 2 Drawing of a midsagittal section through the head showing the brain stem, cerebellum, hippocampus, thalamus, and amygdala. The hippocampus is located on the interior and medial aspect of the temporal lobe. The hippocampus has been implicated in emotional processing and memory. The thalamus serves as the gateway to the cortex for the sensory systems, and the hypothalamus regulates bodily changes like heart rate and temperature. The frontal cortex, especially the medial prefrontal and orbitofrontal cortex, plays a critical role in the regulation of emotion and memory.

tor that reconciles immediately present cognitive-emotional data in the orbitoprefrontal cortex with internal data to effectively activate working emotional sets. This leads to cognitive-emotional control of behavior (Wall & Messier, 2001).

Memory is state-dependent in that there is a relationship between encoding cues and retrieval cues. Understanding that retrieval is a reconstructive process, not a replica of experience, is of significant import for psychotherapy (Pally, 1997). With immaturity of the hippocampus in early childhood, elaborations, errors, and affect-laden insertions are more likely. Retelling the narrative of events in psychotherapy may lead to a modification of the memory. This more elaborate encoding may be effective in enhancing explicit memory (Pally, 1997). Clarification and interpretation in psychotherapy may be an important procedure in modifying the potency of complicated cues to elicit both the overelaborated memory and its associated viscero-emotional component.

THE ROLE OF THE AMYGDALA IN EMOTIONAL MEMORY AND EMOTIONAL PROCESSING

In psychotherapy, the emotions and memories of briefly experienced events are often evoked. Recollections and reminiscences may be elaborated and narratives formed, especially from those experiences having an adverse or overstimulating impact. The significance of experience and the strength of memory depend upon *emotional activation* through neuromodulatory systems involving the amygdaloid complex (AC; Cahill et al., 1996). The AC affects memory through its influences on the hippocampus. This influence, in turn, leads to modifications and feedback to the prefrontal and sensory cortices where consolidation may take place. *Emotional memory*, most often out of awareness, is mediated by amygdala activation, thresholds, and encoded information. The amygdala receives and evaluates the emotional stimulus and sits at the intersection of the input and output systems of fear. Thus, it plays a critical role in processing fear as well as in establishing conditioned responses to the stimuli that evoke it (Bechara et al., 1995; LeDoux, 2002). The amygdala is the key to understanding how "danger" is processed by the brain (LeDoux, 2002).

Sounds that arouse fear reach the lateral amygdala through the thalamus and cortex. These are relayed to the brain stem and hypothalamus through synaptic connections that are modulated by GABA and other neurotransmitters that mediate the fear response. The ability of the amygdala to serve as an interface between threatening stimuli in the environment and defense responses stems from its connections to sensory processing systems and motor control regions (LeDoux, 2002).

Evaluating the context of danger is believed to involve interactions between the hippocampus and amygdala. The basal amygdala—essential in contextual conditioning—receives information processed from the hippocampus through pathways originating in the rhinal areas of the cortex (Fanselow, 1994; Fanselow & Kim, 1994; Fanselow & LeDoux, 1999; Phillips & LeDoux, 1992). This contextual dimension adds a psychological component (associated triggers, state-specific memory cues) of critical importance to our understanding of anxiety and the spectrum of defenses and avoidant behaviors it provokes over time.

The amygdala interacts with the prefrontal cortex (including anterior cingulate and orbital regions) and transitional areas (intralimbic and prelimbic cortex). These areas send connections to several amygdala regions and to the brain stem, allowing cognitive functions organized in the prefrontal regions to regulate the amygdala and its fear reactions. The amygdala and prefrontal cortex are inversely related. Activation of prefrontal cortex inhibits the amygdala, making it harder to express fear (LeDoux, 2002).

Behavioral dispositions reflect functional aspects of systems that are involved in the regulation of behavior and emotional states. For example, behavioral inhibitions may entail activity in fear circuits. Anxiety may involve an attentional bias toward threat cue and a heightened startle reaction, as seen in postramatic stress disorder (PTSD) (Carter, 2001; Kagan, 1995).

A recent study (Cahill et al., 1996; Cahill & McGaugh, 1998; Cahill et al., 1999; Cahill, Haier, & White, 2001) and follow-up data utilizing positron emission tomography (PET) investigated the activity of the AC in the storage of long-term memory for emotionally arousing events. Subjects underwent PET measurements of brain activity while viewing film clips of neutral and emotionally arousing documentaries. (See Figure 3.) Enhanced recall of long-term memory was correlated with increased glucose metabolism in the right AC for the emotional versus the neutral films. The AC demonstrated a selective role in learning and memory processing. Its activation during emotional experiences may be related to long-term conscious recall of these specific experiences. The AC appears to modulate memory storage during periods of emotionally influenced conscious recall. Therefore, when patients are requested to recall emotionally charged memories, they are stimulating their amygdalas. When, during the course of psychotherapy, they are asked to learn or change emotionally charged concepts or perspectives, their amygdalas are activated.

Recent evidence indicates that the amygdala modulates the separate types of memory mediated by the hippocampus and the caudate nucleus. Recent human brain imaging studies also point to both sex- and hemisphere-related asymmetries in amygdala participation in emotionally influenced memory (Packard & Cahill, 2001). An MRI study of caudate nucleus volume in medication-naïve patients with schizotypal personality disorder demonstrated reduced size (similar to neuroleptic-naïve first-episode schizophrenic patients) compared to control subjects. This supports a possible intrinsic pathology in the caudate nucleus, leading to abnormalities in working memory (Levitt et al., 2002).

Amygdala activation reflects moment-to-moment subjective emotional experience. This activation enhances memory in relation to the emotional intensity of the experience (Canli, Zhao, Brewer, Gabrieli, & Cahill, 2000). In males, stimulation of the noradrenergic system results in the enhancement of recall and recognition of the emotional material (O'Carroll, Drysdale, Cahill, Shajahan, & Ebmeier, 1999).

An emerging model of PTSD posits a "duel representation theory" that involves separate memory systems underlying the vivid reexperiencing versus ordinary autobiographical memories of trauma (Brewin, 2001).

The significance of heightened emotion in the consolidation of memory data is a complex matter. Explicit and implicit memories are processed differently and can become disconnected. In the infant, the basal ganglia and amygdala are sufficiently developed to encode memories of an implicit type (movements, experiences, relationship cues) while immaturity of the hippocampus may partially explain childhood "amnesia" for explicit recollections.

Amygdala Complex Activation and Recall of Emotion vs. Neutral Films

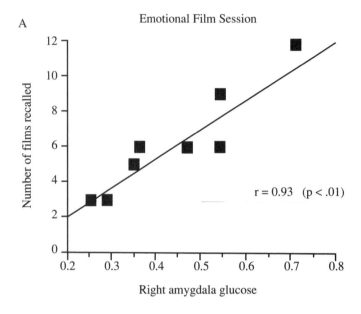

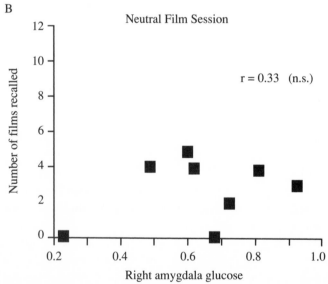

FIGURE 3 Scatterplots of right amygdalid complex glucose metabolism (AC) relative versus recall for both the E and N sessions. (A) Plot of relative glucose metabolism in the right AC during the E session and the number of E films recalled by each subject. (B) The same analysis for the N Session.

When the hippocampus comes "online" at about 18 months, the child's increasing narrative experiences (bedtime dialogue, stories, retelling experiences) and active language acquisition increase childhood explicit memory (Pally, 1997; Siegal, 1996). (Perhaps this is an antecedent and early model for the journaling and self-assessment that is part of cognitive-behavioral psychotherapy.)

Freud and later investigators such as Rappaport were inspired by their clinical observations to view a substantial portion of psychological defenses and reaction patterns as being determined by the complex relationship between emotions and memory (Rappaport, 1942, 1953, 1967; Freud, 1950/1966b, 1936/1964).

Under mild stress, there may be an increase in orienting, alerting, and focusing systems to enhance recall. Severe traumatic stress, however, may lead to dissociated implicit/explicit recall with remembrance of only isolated segments of an event or selected elements of the associated emotional-visceral reactions. Flashbacks (sudden reliving of past events) may be memories of traumatic events without a hippocampal location/time marker, an absence that leads to a flooded or intrusive disruption of ambient functioning. In the startle and hyper-alert sequelae of trauma, there is an activation of the amygdala without explicit recall. Psychotherapy may facilitate explicit processing of trauma by reestablishing perspective (locations and time markers, enhancing hippocampal function) and contrasting and comparing past events with current experiences through contemporary narratives (Pally 1997b). In the most severe and chronic experiences of trauma, actual hippocampal atrophy may restrict attempts to treat and anticipate change (Bremner, 1995).

Events or aspects of events in our daily life not only may be processed by separate memory systems, but also can be activated or recalled separately under certain conditions (Schacter, 1992; Schacter et al., 1996). A PET study demonstrated that if subjects identified a word as one they thought they had heard previously, there was activity in the hippocampus; if the word had actually been heard and remembered, activity was found in both the auditory cortex and hippocampus; if the word was only "remembered," activity was in the hippocampus alone. The activity of the hippocampus may contribute a sense of veracity to memory (Schacter, 1996, 2001; Dodson, Koutstaal, & Schacter, 2000).

The human amygdala is capable of undergoing emotional learning from stimuli that are never experienced in full awareness. For example, unconscious emotional learning may occur directly from sensory areas (thalamus) to the amygdala without involving the neocortex (Morris, Ohman, & Dolan, 1998, 1999). Damage to the amygdala interferes with the ability to judge emotions expressed in faces and voices and appears to interfere with the development of basic trust in others (Adolphs, Tranel, & Damasio, 1998; Breiter, Etcoff, et al., 1996; Breiter, Rauch, & Kwong, 1996; Morris et al., 1996; Whalen et al., 1998).

Nondeclarative memory (procedural, emotional) takes place below awareness and encodes information that mediates motor skills, routine actions, cognitive orientations, and emotional responses. The basal ganglia integrates procedural information and may have a role in habitual modes of action embodied in our character traits. The amygdala is central in integrating and modulating emotional memory.

Clinically, repression is manifested as explicit memory blocked from full awareness, possibly due to an inhibitory (conflictual, negative) affect associated with information stored in long-term memory. The right frontal lobe may function to prevent/screen painful memories from gaining access to the left hemisphere, where overintensive analysis may occur (Joseph, 1996).

In psychotherapy, clues to implicit encoded experience may manifest themselves through the therapist's experience of transient reveries, empathic resonance with the patient, nonverbal cues (speech, tone, facial expression, movements) and therapist countertransference experiences (Pally, 1997b). Often there will be a spurt of clinical progress (e.g., symptom reduction, a positive change in affect, diminished resistance to psychotherapy) when implicit memory expressions (procedural and emotional) are reconnected to explicit details of events (Pally, 1997b).

The declarative, procedural, and emotional learning systems organize the ability to adapt to the interpersonal field as well as to the material environment. What we individuals know about and do with one another, as well as how emotions play a role in an individual's behavioral repertoire, rely upon and utilize the brain's multiple memory systems.

Knowledge of how these dissociable memory systems function provides a novel perspective on relationships—both ordinary social relationships and those that develop in psychotherapy—and further illuminates psychotherapeutic transference and counter-transference phenomena (Grigsby & Stevens, 2002). The search for the neurobiologic underpinnings of mental processes gives hope for increasing diagnostic clarity and therapeutic effectiveness.

The challenges to understanding unconscious mental processes include: the nature of psychological causality (a guiding principle in psychoanalysis/psychodynamic theory), developmental psychopathology, the role of early experience, structural and functional changes in the brain as a result of psychotherapy, and the integration of psychotherapy and pharmacotherapy (for specific diagnostic disorders and for the enhancement of learning) (Kandel, 1999a, 1999b).

NEUROBIOLOGIC SUBSTRATES FOR THERAPEUTIC CHANGE

Psychotherapeutic transformation in the brain may be mediated by three fundamental processes that over time continue to be elaborated by theory and research. First is *the formation of new structures* (e.g., constructivism; see Quartz & Sejnowski, 1997) through axonal/dendritic growth and complexity. The extent of human postnatal cortical development in building mental representations under the guidance of the environment has been widely underestimated. The "Constructivist Manifesto" argues that (1) learning guides brain development and leads to major changes in the underlying brain hardware, (2) representational structures are progressively added during development, and (3) the sets, processes, and structures that transform imputed data into a *steady state* are *nonstationary*. Candidates that may serve as complexity measures include increased synaptic numbers, dendritic arborization, and axonal arborization.

Mechanisms in neuronal learning and memory are not only used and revised in structuring the central nervous system during the initial establishment of connections in the immature brain, but also can be employed in molding personality and behavior during psychotherapy in adulthood (Braun & Bogerts, 2001).

Second is *synaptic plasticity* (Kandel, 1999a; Lüscher, 2000; Zucker, 1999), a main factor in ambient and enduring change in the central nervous system. Through the effect of experience upon neuronal reactivity, chemical and structural modifications that alter nerve conduction at critical and multiple junctions (long-term potentiation) are induced. This results in sensitization, facilitation, inhibition, and extinction of responsivity. The hippocampus (dentate, A1 and C3 regions), prefrontal cortex, and amygdala are crucial sites where emotional, memory, behavioral integration, and processing take place. The induction of gene expression altering synthesis of critical enzymes underlies the encoding and decoding process.

Third is *contemporary addition*. This occurs through neurogenesis, which may underlie and enhance critical points in the temporal neuronal encoding of experience (Gould et al., 1999; Manev, H., 2001; Manev, R., 2001; Shors et al., 2001; Van Praag et al., 2002). Trace memories depend on hippocampal neurogenesis (Shors, Miesegaes, Beylin, Zhao, Rydel, & Gould, 2001). Neurogenesis in the adult hippocampus leads to additional functioning neurons (Van Praag, 2002). From birth to 3 months, the total cortical number of neurons increases 27%. Subsequently, from 3 to 24 months, it decreases back to its birth value. Then, from months 24 to 72, it increases by 69–90% (Shankle, Landing, Hara, & Fallon, 1998). (See Figure 4.)

The preceding constructional anlage and the gradual accumulation of a knowledge base derived from genetic and imaging studies in cognitive neuroscience can form the neurobiologic foundation of a psychotherapy science.

NEURAL BASES OF EXECUTIVE FUNCTIONING

The effects of emotion on executive function (the set of cognitive operations required to maintain organized information and coordinated actions of the brain) may play an important role in the nonadaptive, nonerror-correcting behavior common to enduring mental conflict. Cognitive central mechanisms, such as an "attentional set" guide the processing of information in a task-appropriate manner. Evaluative processes monitor for evidence of poor performance, such as response conflict, and signal when stronger control needs to be engaged (Carter, 2001).

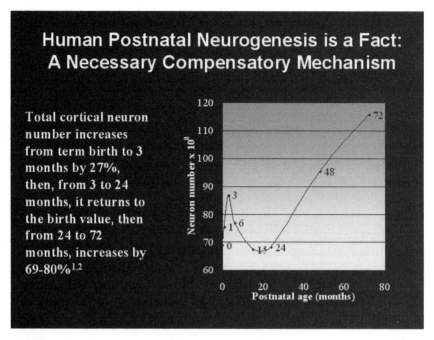

FIGURE 4 Total number of neurons in human cerebral cortex: Birth to 72 months. The total cortical neuron number increases from term birth to 3 months by 27.9%; then from 3–24 months it returns to the birth value; then from 24–72 months it increases by 69–80% (Shankle, Landing, Hara, & Fallon, 1998). (Reproduced with permission.)

The frontal lobes (the anterior cingulate cortex [ACC] and the dorsolateral prefrontal cortex [DLPFC] play a central role in executive function. The ACC receives rich projections from the amygdala and has broad output throughout the motor system, thus supporting its significant role in behavioral control (D'Esposito, Detre, & Alsop, 1995; Mesulam, 1980). The ACC is involved in error detection and compensation; this region of the brain detects conflicts and is part of an error-prevention network that triggers strategic processing in the service of conflict resolution (Carter, 2001). Indicative of the DLPFC's "top-down" control is its association of increased activity with representations of context and the maintenance of an attentional set. The ACC, on the other hand, evaluates the level of response conflict and signals when control needs to be more strongly engaged (Carter, 2001). (See Figure 5.)

Executive Functions: Attention Set, Reponse, Conflict, Error Correction

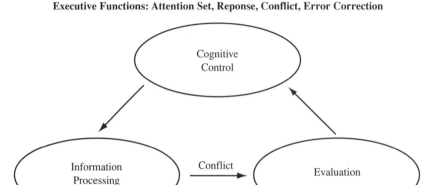

FIGURE 5 A schematic model of executive functions as a set of dynamic processes. Cognitive control mechanisms, such as attentional set, bias information processing in a task-appropriate manner. Evaluative processes monitor for evidence of poor performance, such as response conlict, and signal when control needs to be more strongly engaged (Carter, 2001). (Used by permission.)

In obsessive-compulsive disorder (OCD), hyperactivity of the ACC may provide the individual with a faulty appraisal of his or her own functioning and an inappropriate sense that corrective actions need to be taken even during a normative situation.

In psychotherapy, awareness of the neural bases of clinical symptoms and possible mechanisms of action for treatment (pharmacotherapeutic modification or psychotherapeutic intervention) can aid in gauging both the intensity of therapeutic effort and realistic expectations of results. For example, Breiter, Rauch, and Kwong (1996) demonstrated increased limbic system activation (amygdala, orbitofrontal, and cingulate cortices) in OCD by exposing subjects to stimuli specific to their individual obsessions or compulsions.

ABNORMAL EMOTIONAL FUNCTIONING IN AFFECTIVE AND ANXIETY DISORDERS

Specific brain regions may be involved in the recognition of emotion in the external world (George & Ketter, 1997). Responsivity to emotion in the human face is diminished in depressed patients. For example, PET studies have demonstrated decreased activation bilaterally in temporal lobes and in the right insular area in depressed patients compared to normal controls. The emotional recognition deficit in depression resembles deficits found in persons with focal right hemisphere brain damage. Abnormal function of limbic and immediately adjacent regions may partially explain these facial emotion recognition deficits. Implications for effects on empathy and social interaction in the depressed individual are clear. The neurobiologic deficit may initiate and amplify both intrapsychic and interpersonal conflict during a depressive episode. In persistent dysthymic disorders it may blunt the affective reciprocity needed to initiate and maintain intimate and family relationships. In psychotherapy, therapists may provide a useful perspective by helping the patient to understand the inhibitions of this crucial empathic capacity and to appreciate what may be missed in his or her interpretations of relationships and understanding the reactions of family members. One may also consider devising procedures that promote small steps of stimulation and interaction. Thus, an understanding of the brain pathology of affective illness and the basis for the potential psychosocial conflict that may follow is enhanced.

Male patients with first-episode major depression had significantly smaller hippocampal total and gray-matter volumes than healthy male comparison subjects. These findings support the hypothesis that the hippocampus and its connections within the limbic-cortical networks may play a crucial role in the pathogenesis of major depression (Frodl et al., 2002). Genetic and animal model studies suggest that small hippocampal size may be a genetic risk factor for (rather than a consequence of) depression. Once a mood disorder is initiated, complex stress-hormonal, neuroimmune, and environmental factors may magnify neurocognitive impairment (especially problems of focus and encoding dependent on prefrontal/anterior cingulated-hippocampal connections) and trigger a cascade of cardiovascular casualty (clotting abnormalities, arrhythmias) and early mortality (Schatzberg, 2002).

The processing of emotionally salient faces may stimulate simultaneous recruitment of the amygdala and ventral temporal regions. Differences in amygdala activation when stimulated by evocative faces have been found when comparing healthy to over-anxious adolescents and adults (Pine, 2001). Face-processing studies have revealed a memory bias toward hostile faces in social phobia and a hypervigilence for angry faces in anxiety disorders (Mogg & Bradly, 1999). Imaging studies may help to define attentional and memory processes significant in human object relations. These have implications for psychotherapy.

Neuroscience has disclosed that attachment is a complex neurobiologic phenomenon mediated by specific brain structures (orbitofrontal cortex) and neurochemical modulations (opioid mediation of separation distress and the role of benzodiazapine receptors in the amygdala). Attachment functions as a biological regulator of multiple systems (affect, feeding, growth, and mating) (Panksepp, 1998; Schore, 1994; Kalin, Shelton, & Lynn, 1995; Davis, 1992; Blinder, Chaitin, & Goldstein, 1988).

A recent PET study comparing bulimia nervosa patients to normal controls demonstrated remarkable caudate hypermetabolism and increased activity in amygdala and cingulate areas of the brain in patients with bulimia nervosa. (Klein, Blinder, & Wu, 1996). Prior PET studies had shown bulimia nervosa to have a classic asymmetric (left side greater than right) glucose metabolic activity that was distinct from the patterns observed in depression. (Hagman et al., 1990; Wu et al., 1990). The finding of pronounced activity in the caudate area suggests a neurobiological basis relating eating disorders to the basal ganglia-cingulate-frontal lobe *worry circuit* in obsessive-compulsive disorders. Through evolution the caudate area has come to connect food seeking and food preparatory behavior.

A significant group of studies have defined an important role for dopaminergic/serotonergic and possibly other neurotransmitter determinants of both regulatory and instrumental components of feeding. In the caudate nucleus of the basal ganglia, these feeding components involve consummatory behavior, aphagia/hyperphagia, food seeking, and reactions to the visualization of food. The basal ganglia may function primarily as an alerting and sensorimotor integrator for feeding/consummatory preparation, pursuit, and termination. This motor behavior with feeding is in contrast to appetite satiety regulation in the hypothalamus.

Many of the obsessional and ritual behaviors in eating disorders that resist modification and therapeutic intervention may be driven by the foregoing neurobiologic mechanisms. We have learned that gradual cognitive-behavioral and nutritional rehabilitative approaches are necessary in the initial phases of treatment of eating disorders. More extensive psychodynamic psychotherapy addressing developmental conflict is often best applied at a later point in the course of a comprehensive therapeutic approach. A developmental psychopathology of the eating disorder is gradually emerging from observation and research into the developmental stages of feeding, attachment and separation, and the psychobiology of appetite regulation and food selection (Blinder, 1988).

A PET study of reactions to phobogenic and anxiety-provoking stimuli distinguished different regions of the brain involved in anxiety and phobic responses (Fredrickson et al., 1993; Wik et al., 1993). Visually induced fear and anxiety were associated with alterations in limbic, paralimbic, and cortical brain regions.

The specific phobic response (snake/spiders) demonstrated the functional neuroanatomy of a visually elicited *defense reaction* with activation in *secondary* but not *primary* visual areas and *deactivation* in the hippocampus, prefrontal, orbitofrontal, and posterior cingulate areas. The amygdala was normally reactive.

The activation of the visual association cortex is seen in generalized anxiety disorder (GAD), OCD, and panic disorder and suggests that hypervigilence is a common characteristic associated with fear and anxiety. The paralimbic and frontal reduction in activity reflect behavioral inhibition and decreased cognitive processing associated with a defense reaction. Decreased neural activity in the orbitofrontal region during anxiety may facilitate the initiation and direction of attention for action. This neurobiologic substrate of *defense* parallels the understanding derived from naturalistic observations of clinical states and psychotherapeutic processes.

EMOTIONAL PROCESSING IN DREAMS: AN INTERPLAY OF VISUAL, LIMBIC, AND CORTICAL REGIONS

A comparison was made between the REM (rapid eye movement) sleep and the waking PET scans of ten healthy male volunteers to evaluate regional interrelationships within visual cortices and their projections during REM sleep in human subjects. REM sleep was found to be associated with activation of the extrastriate visual cortices with attenuated activity in the primary visual cortex (Braun et al., 1998). Additionally, the activity of the extrastriates was associated with concomitant activation of the limbic and adjacent regions, with reduced activity in the frontal association areas.

These findings suggest that the visual and limbic areas operate actively during dreaming sleep (REM) and operate functionally as a closed system, one that is disconnected from the frontal lobes. This dissociation may explain many experiential dream features such as heightened emotionality, uncritical acceptance of bizarre content, parallel thoughts and images, temporal distortions, and the absence of reflective awareness. The "primary process" mental functioning in dreams suggested by Freud is certainly elicited, although views about the presence of more complex cognition during sleep may need to be modified. The interpretation of dreams may be more significant as a clue to affective states (anxiety, panic, depression, aggression) than for more elaborate cognitive meanings. The significance of "dream work" in problem-solving, transference, and complex psychological defenses will need reinvestigation and reinterpretation in psychotherapy. However, the correlation of dream content with brain function will present further methodologic and interpretive challenges.

Systematic explorations of the experiential recovered content of dreams suggest specific localization of brain metabolic activity associated with anxiety and aggression as both perceived affect and enacted behavior (Gottschalk et al., 1991). The role of dreams in psychotherapy is clearly multidetermined. Dreams may have both a communication/disclosure function and a neurobiologic consolidation outcome that aid in processing experience.

PSYCHOTHERAPEUTIC AND PHARMACOLOGIC CHANGE: A COMMON NEUROLOGICAL LANGUAGE

Kandel (1998) proposed a common framework for psychiatry and the neural sciences: (1) all mental processes derive from the brain, (2) genes and their protein products (neurohormones) determine neuronal connections and functioning, (3) learning can produce alterations in gene expression and psychosocial factors feed back to the brain, (4) altered gene expression in response to learning changes neuronal connections that contribute to individuality and maintaining abnormalities of behavior, and (5) psychotherapy produces long-term behavior change by altering gene expression, yielding structural changes in the brain.

Gradual changes in affect, insight, motivation, and behavior resulting from the psychotherapeutic processes and technical procedures are reflected in modifications in neural structure. Treatments that change behavior may do so by producing alterations in gene expression, which, in turn, produce new structural changes in the brain. Both pharmacological intervention and psychotherapy in the treatment of "neuroses" should, if successful, produce functional and structural change. Brain-imaging studies in the future may aid in diagnosing enduring conflict states and in assessing the progress of psychotherapy. Pharmacotherapy and psychotherapy may be synergistic for change by promoting consolidation of the biological substrate of their individual and combined effects.

Antianxiety, antidepressive, and antischizophrenic medications have been shown in neuropsychopharmacologic studies to significantly decrease the magnitude of verbal content-analysis derived scores for anxiety, depression, and the schizophrenic syndrome in the appropriate and expected direction (Gottschalk, 1999, 2002).

Recent studies (Brody & Saxena, 2001; Furmark et al., 2002; Martin & Martin, 2001) have shown similar normalizing brain changes in the treatment of depression and social phobia with either antidepressants (paroxaetine, venlafaxine, citalopram) or interpersonal psychotherapy and cognitive behavioral therapy. Despite methodological limitations, there was indication that antidepressants and psychotherapy may act on similar systems selectively in exerting therapeutic action. In other words, changes in functional brain activity following pharmacotherapy and psychotherapy were remarkably similar. Psychotherapy as a learning experience may lead to changes in synaptic plasticity through a retraining of the implicit memory systems. Because prior studies have found a poor response to psychotherapy in cohorts of depressed patients with increased limbic activity on PET scans, pharmacotherapy may be more effective in this subgroup by virtue of more direct effects on neural circuits or gene activity (Sackheim, 2001; Thase, 2001). Variations such as length and frequency of sessions, use of participation and arousal techniques, and awareness of stereotyped resistances in cognitive sets and behavior may be linked to a rational neurobiologic understanding. However, there needs to be more understanding of how the brain changes during acquisition of information, what processes are involved in learning that information and how the learned information affects future behavior. From paradigms of conditioning to more complex models of learning, we now seek to understand and capture the indicators of change in the central nervous system that reflect the alterations in behavior and meaning that signify clinical improvement and gains in adaptation and human potential.

Naturalistic observations of psychopathology in behavior, affect, relationships, and interpretations of the course and nature of psychotherapy are extended and amplified by knowledge gained from neurobiologic studies. Freud's descriptions of the psychopathology of everyday life, patterns of neurotic behavior, symptomatic behaviors, and dreams are now given new meaning, with hope for greater understanding and possibilities for transformations through the use of new and enlightened treatments.

References

Adolphs, R., Tranel, D., & Damasio, A. R. (1998). The human amygdala in social judgement. *Nature, 393,* 470–474.

Adolphs, R., Tranel, D., Damasio, H., & Damasio, A. R. (1994). Impaired recognition of emotion in facial expressions following bilateral damage to the amygdala. *Nature, 372,* 669–672.

Agras, W. S., Rossiter, E. M., Arnow, B., Schneider, J. A., Telch, C. F., Raeburn, S. D., et al. (1992). Pharmacologic and cognitive-behavioral treatment for bulimia nervosa: A controlled comparison. *American Journal of Psychiatry, 149,* 82–87.

Alexander, G. E., DeLong, M. R., & Strick P. L. (1986). Parallel organization of functionally segregated circuits linking basal ganglia and cortex. *Annual Review of Neuroscience, 9,* 357–381.

American Medical Association Council on Ethical and Judicial Affairs. (1999). *Code of medical ethics: Current opinions with annotations.* Washington, DC: Author.

American Psychiatric Association. (1980). Guidelines for psychiatrists in consultative, supervisory, or collaborative relationships with nonmedical therapists. *American Journal of Psychiatry, 137,* 1489–1491.

American Psychiatric Association. (1994). *Diagnostic and statistical manual of mental disorders (4th ed.)* Washington, DC: Author.

American Psychiatric Association. (1997a). Practice guidelines for the treatment of patients with schizophrenia. *American Journal of Psychiatry, 154* (Suppl. 4), 1–63.

American Psychiatric Association. (1997b). *Principles of medical ethics with annotations especially applicable to psychiatry.* Washington, DC: Author.

American Psychiatric Association. (1998). Practice guidelines for the treatment of patients with panic disorder. *American Journal of Psychiatry, 155* (Suppl. 5), 1–34.

American Psychiatric Association. (1993). Practice guideline for major depressive disorder in adults. *American Journal of Psychiatry, 150* (Suppl. 4), 1–26.

Angst, J., Sellaro, R., & Merikangas, K. R. (2000). Depressive spectrum diagnoses. *Comprehensive Psychiatry, 41,* 39–47.

Appelbaum, P. S. (1991). General guidelines for psychiatrists who prescribe medication for patients treated by nonmedical psychotherapists. *Hospital and Community Psychiatry, 43,* 281–282.

Baggs, J. G., & Schmitt, M. H. (1988). Collaboration between nurses and physicians. *Journal Nursing Scholarship, 20,* 145–149.

Ballenger, J. C., Davidson, J. R. T., Lecrubier,Y., Nutt, D. J., Baldwin, D. S., Den Boer, J. A., et al. (1998). Consensus statement on panic disorder from the International Consensus Group on Depression and Anxiety. *Journal of Clinical Psychiatry, 59* (Suppl. 8), 47–54.

Balon, R. (1999). Positive aspects of collaborative treatment. In M. B. Riba & R. Balon (Eds.), *Psychopharmacology and psychotherapy: A collaborative approach* (pp. 1–31). Washington, DC: American Psychiatric Press.

Barden, N., Reul, J. M. H. M., & Holsboer, F. (1995). Do antidepressants stabilize mood through actions on the hypothalamic-pituitary-adrenocortical system? *Trends in Neuroscience, 18,* 6–11.

Barlow, D. H., Gorman, J. M., Shear, M. K., & Woods, S. W. (2000). Cognitive-behavioral therapy, imipramine, or their combination for panic disorder: A randomized controlled trial. JAMA, *283,* 2529–2536.

Baron-Cohen, S., Ring, H., Moriatry, J., Schmitz, B., Costa, D., & Ell, P. (1994). Recognition of mental state terms: Clinical findings in children with autism and a functional neuroimaging study of normal adults. *British Journal of Psychiatry, 165,* 640–649.

Basco, M. R., & Rush, A. J. (1995). Compliance of pharmacotherapy in mood disorders. *Psychiatric Annals, 25,* 269–270, 276–279.

Basco, M. R., & Rush, A. J. (1996). *Cognitive-behavioral therapy for bipolar disorder.* New York: Guilford.

Bascue, L. O., & Zlotowski, M. (1980). Psychologists' practices related to medication. *Journal of Clinical Psychology, 36,* 821–825.

Basoglu, M., Marks, I. M., Kilic, C., Brewin, C. R., & Swinson, R. P. (1994). Alprazolam and exposure for panic disorder with agoraphobia: Attribution of improvement of medication predicts subsequent relapse. *British Journal of Psychiatry, 164,* 652–659.

Basoglu, M., Marks, I. M., Swinson, R. P., Noshirvani, H., O'Sullivan, G., & Kuch, K. (1994). Pre-treatment predictors of treatment outcome in panic disorder and agoraphobia treated with alprazolam and exposure. *Journal of Affective Disorders, 30,* 123–132.

Baxter, L. R., Schwartz, J. M., Bergman, K. S., Szuba, M. P., Guze, B. H., Mazziotta, et al. (1992). Caudate glucose metabolic rate changes with both drug and behavior therapy for obsessive-compulsive disorder. *Archives of General Psychiatry, 49,* 681–690.

Beach S., Sandeen, E., & O'Leary, K. (1990). *Depression in marriage.* New York: Guilford.

Beaudry, P. (1991). Generalized anxiety disorder. In B. D. Beitman, & G. L. Klerman (Eds.), *Integrating pharmacotherapy and psychotherapy* (pp. 211–230). Washington, DC: American Psychiatric Press.

Bechara, A., Tranel, D., Damasio, H., Adolphs, R., Rockland, C., & Damasio, A. R. (1995). Double dissociation of conditioning and declarative knowledge relative to the amygdala and hippocampus in humans. *Science, 269* (5227), 1115–1118.

Beck, A. T. (1976). *Cognitive therapy and the emotional disorders.* New York: International Universities Press.

Beck, A. T., Hollon, S. D., Young, J. F., Bedrosian, R. C., & Budenz, D. (1985). Treatment of depression with cognitive therapy and amitriptyline. *Archives of General Psychiatry, 42,* 142–148.

Beck, A. T., Ward, C. H., Mendelson, M., Mack, J., & Erbaugh, J. (1961). An inventory for measuring depression. *Archives of General Psychiatry, 4,* 561–571.

Beck, J. S. (2001). A cognitive therapy approach to medication compliance. In J. Kay (Ed.), *Integrated treatment of psychiatric disorders* (pp. 113–140). Washington, DC: American Psychiatric Publishing.

Beitman, B. D. (1983). The demographics of American psychotherapists: A pilot study. *American Journal of Psychiatry, 37*, 37–48.

Beitman, B. D. (1993). Pharmacotherapy and the stages of psychotherapeutic change. In J. M. Oldham, M. B. Riba, & H. Tasman (Eds.), *Review of Psychiatry, 12*. Washington, DC: American Psychiatric Press.

Beitman, B. D., Beck, N. C., Deuser, W. E., Carter, C. S., Davidson, J. R. T., & Maddock, R. I. (1994). Patient stage of change predicts outcome in a panic disorder medication trial. *Anxiety, 1,* 64–69.

Beitman, B. D., Chiles, J., & Carlin, A. (1984). The pharmacotherapy-psychotherapy triangle: Psychiatrist, nonmedical psychotherapist, and patient. *Journal of Clinical Psychiatry, 45,* 458–459.

Beitman, B. D., Hall, M. J., & Woodward, B. (1992). Integrating pharmacotherapy and psychotherapy. In J. C. Norcross & M. R. Goldfried (Eds.), *Handbook of psychotherapy integration* (pp. 533–562). New York: Basic Books.

Beitman, B. D., & Klerman, G. L. (1991). *Integrating pharmacotherapy and psychotherapy.* Washington, DC: American Psychiatric Press.

Beitman, B. D., & Yue D. (1999). *Learning psychotherapy.* New York: Norton.

Benton, M. K., & Schroeder, H. E. (1990). Social skills training with schizophrenics: A meta-analytic evaluation. *Journal of Consulting and Clinical Psychology, 58,* 741–747.

Blackburn, I. M., Bishop, S., Glen, A. I. M., Whalley, L. J., & Christie, J. E. (1981). The efficacy of cognitive therapy in depression: A treatment trial using cognitive therapy and pharmacotherapy, each alone and in combination. *British Journal of Psychiatry, 139,* 181–189.

Blinder, B. J., Chaitin, B. F., & Goldstein, R. (1988). *The eating disorders: Medical and psychological bases of diagnosis and treatment.* New York: PMA Publications.

Blomhoff, S., Haug, Hellström, K., Holme, I., Humble, M., Madsbu, H. P., & Wold, J. E. (2001). Randomised controlled general practice trial of sertraline, exposure therapy and combined treatment in generalized social phobia. *British Journal of Psychiatry, 179*, 23–30.

Bowers, W. A. (1990). Treatment of depressed in-patients: Cognitive therapy plus medication, relaxation plus medication, and medication alone. *British Journal of Psychiatry, 156*, 73–78.

Bradley, S. J. (2000). *Affect regulation and the development of psychopathology.* New York: Guilford.

Bradley, S. S. (1990). Nonphysician psychotherapist-physician pharmacotherapist: A new model for concurrent treatment. *Psychiatric Clinics of North America, 13*, 307–322.

Braun, A. R., Balkin, T. J., Wesensten, N. J., Gwadry, F., Carson, R. E., Varga, M., Baldwin, P., Belenky, G., & Herscovitch, P. (1998). Dissociated pattern of activity in visual cortices and their projections during human rapid eye movement sleep. *Science, 279*, 91–95.

Braun, K., & Bogerts, B. (2001). Experience guided neuronal plasticity: Significance for pathogenesis and therapy of psychiatric diseases. *Nervenarzt, 72*(1), 3–10.

Breiter, H. C., Etcoff, N. L., Whalen, P. J., Kennedy, W. A., Rauch, S. L., Buchner, R. L., et al. (1996). Response and habituation of the human amygdala during visual processing of facial expression. *Neuron, 17*, 875–887.

Breiter, H. C., Rauch, S. L., & Kwong, K. K. (1996). Functional magnetic resonance imaging of symptom provocation in obsessive compulsive disorder. *Archives of General Psychiatry, 53*, 595–606.

Bremner, J. D., Krystal, J. H., Southwick, S. M., & Charney, D. S. (1995). Functional neuroanatonical correlates of the effects of stress on memory. *Journal of Trauma Stress, 8*(4), 527–553.

Bremner, J. D., Randall, P., Scott, T. M., Bronen, R. A., Seibyl, J. P., Southwick, S. M., et al. (1995). MRI-based measurement of hippocampal volume in patients with combat-related posttraumatic stress disorder. *American Journal of Psychiatry, 152*, 973–981.

Brewin, C. R. (2001). A cognitive neuroscience account of posttraumatic stress disorder and its treatment. *Behavior Research & Therapy, 39*(4), 373–393.

Brody, A. L., & Saxena, S. (2001). Regional brain metabolic changes in patients with major depression treated with either

Paroxetine or interpersonal therapy. *Archives of General Psychiatry, 58,* 631–640.

Brown, G. W., Birley, J. L. T., & Wing, J. K. (1972). Influence of family life on the course of schizophrenic disorders: A replication. *British Journal of Psychiatry, 121,* 241–258.

Busch, F. N., & Gould, E. (1993). Treatment by a psychotherapist and a psychopharmacologist: Transference and countertransference issues. *Hospital and Community Psychiatry, 44,* 772–774.

Butzlaff, R. L., & Hooley, J. M. (1998). Expressed emotion and psychiatric relapse: A meta-analysis. *Archives of General Psychiatry, 55,* 547–552.

Caffey, E. M. Jr., Galbrecht, C. R., & Klett, C. J. (1971). Brief hospitalization and aftercare in the treatment of schizophrenia. *Archives of General Psychiatry, 24,* 81–86.

Cahill, L., Haier, R. J., Fallon, J., Alkire, M. T., Tang, C., Keator, D., et al. (1996). Amygdala activity at encoding correlated with long-term, free recall of emotional information. *Proceedings of the National Academy of Science, 93,* 8016–8021.

Cahill, L., Haier, R. J., White, N. S., Fallon, J., Kilpatrick, L., Lawrence, C., et al. (2001). Sex-related differences in amygdala activity during emotionally influenced memory storage. *Neurobiology of Learning and Memory, 75,* 1–9.

Cahill, L., & McGaugh, J. L. (1998). Mechanisms of emotional arousal and lasting declarative memory. *Trends in Neurosciences, 21,* 294–299.

Cahill, L., Weinberger, N. M., Roozendahl, B., & McGaugh, J. L. (1999). Is the amygdala a locus of "conditional fear?" Some questions and caveats. *Neuron, 23,* 227–228.

Canli, T., Zhao, Z., Brewer, J., Gabrieli, J. D., & Cahill, L. (2000). Event-related activation in the human amygdala associates with later memory for individual emotional experience. *Journal of Neuroscience, 20*(19), RC99.

Carroll, B. J. (1991). Psychopathology and neurobiology of manic-depressive disorders. In B. J. Carroll & J. E. Barrett (Eds.), *Psychopathology and the brain* (pp. 265–285). New York: Raven.

Carroll, K. M., Rounsaville, B. J., Gordon, L. T., Nich, C., Jatlow, P., Bisighini,R. M., & et al. (1994). Psychotherapy and pharmacotherapy for ambulatory cocaine abusers. *Archives of General Psychiatry, 51,* 177–187.

Carter, C. S. (2001). *Cognitive Neuroscience: The New Neuroscience of the Mind and Implications for Psychiatry.* In Morisha, J. (ed.). *Advances in brain imaging* (pp. 25–52). Washington: American Psychiatric Publishing, Inc.

Chiles, J. A., Carlin, A. S., Benjamin, G. A. H., & Beitman, B. D. (1991). A physician, a nonmedical psychotherapist, and a patient: The pharmacotherapy-psychotherapy triangle. In B. D. Beitman & G. L. Klerman (Eds.), *Integrating pharmacotherapy and psychotherapy.* Washington, DC: American Psychiatric Press.

Cloninger, C. R., Svrakic, D. M., & Pryzbeck, T. R. (1993). A psychobiological model of temperament and character. *Archives of General Psychiatry, 50,* 975–990.

Cochran, S. D. (1984). Preventing medical noncompliance in the outpatient treatment of bipolar affective disorders. *Journal of Consulting and Clinical Psychology, 52,* 873–878.

Cole, D. P., Thase, M. E., Mallinger, A. G., Soares, J. C., Luther, J. F., Kupfer, D. J., & et al. (2002). Slower treatment response in bipolar depression predicted by lower pretreatment thyroid function. *American Journal of Psychiatry, 159,* 116–121.

Conte, H. R., Plutchik, R., Wild, K. V., & Karasu, T. B. (1986). Combined psychotherapy and pharmacotherapy for depression: A systematic analysis of the evidence. *Archives of General Psychiatry, 43,* 471–479.

Crits-Christoph, P., Siqueland, L., Blaine, J., Frank, A., Luborsky, L., Onken, L., et al. (1999). Psychosocial treatments for cocaine dependence: Results of the National Institute on Drug Abuse collaborative cocaine treatment study. *Archives of General Psychiatry, 56,* 493–502.

Curran, H. V. (1986). Tranquillising memories: A review of the effects of benzodiazepines on human memory. *Biological Psychology, 23,* 179–213.

Damasio, A. (1994). *Descartes' Error.* New York: Grossett/Putnam.

Davis, K. L., Charney, D., Coyle, J. T., & Nemeroff, C. (2002). *Neuropsychopharmacology: The fifth generation of progress.* Philadelphia: Lippincott Williams & Wilkins.

Davis, M. (1992). The role of the amygdala in fear and anxiety. *Annual Review of Neuroscience, 15,* 353–375.

DeBellis, M. D., Gold, P. W., Geracioti, T. D., Listwak, S. J., & Kling, M. A. (1993). Association of fluoxetine treatment with reductions in CSF concentrations of corticotropin-releasing hormone and arginine vasopressin in patients with major depression. *American Journal of Psychiatry, 150,* 656–657.

Depression Guidelines Panel. (1993). Clinical practice guideline number 5. *Depression in primary care, vol 2. Treatment of major depression* (AHCPR Publication No. 93–0551). Rockville, MD: U. S. Department of Health and Human Services Agency for Health Care Policy and Research.

D'Esposito, M., Detre, J., & Alsop, D. (1995). The neural basis of the central executive system of working memory. *Nature, 378,* 279–281.

Dewan, M. (1999). Are psychiatrists cost-effective? An analysis of integrated versus split treatment. *American Journal of Psychiatry, 156*(2), 324–326.

Dicks, D., Myers, R. E., & Kling, A. (1969). Uncus and amygdaloid lesions in social behavior in the free ranging monkey. *Science, 160,* 69–71.

DiMascio, A., Weissman, M. M., Prusoff, B. A., Neu, C., Zwiling, M., & Klerman, G. L. (1979). Differential symptom reduction by drugs and psychotherapy in acute depression. *Archives of General Psychiatry, 36,* 1450–1456.

Dodson, C. S., Koutstaal, W., Schacter, D. L. (2000). Escape for illusion: Reducing false memories. *Trends in Cognitive Science, 4,* 391–397.

Drury, V., Birchwood, M., Cochrane, R., & MacMillan, F. (1996). Cognitive therapy and recovery from acute psychosis: A controlled trial. I. Impact on psychotic symptoms. *British Journal of Psychiatry, 169,* 593–601.

Duffy, J. D., & Campbell, J. J. (1994). The regional prefrontal syndromes: A clinical and theoretical overview. *Journal of Neuropsychiatry and Clinical Neuroscience, 6,* 379–387.

Duffy, F. (2001, May) 1997. Integrated versus split treatments: Pharmacotherapy and psychotherapy for mood disorders. Presented at Commission on Psychotherapy by Psychiatrists, Washington, DC.

Elkin, I., Shea, M. T., Watkins, J. T., Imber, S. D., Sotsky, S. M., Collins, J. F., et al. (1989). National Institute of Mental Health Treatment of Depression Collaborative Research Program: General effectiveness and treatments. *Archives of General Psychiatry, 46,* 971–982.

Epstein N., & Bishop, D. (1992). Problem-centered systems therapy of the family. In A. Gurman & D. Kniskern (Eds.), *Handbook of family therapy* (pp. 444–482). New York: Brunner-Mazel.

Fairburn, C. G., Jones, R., Peveler, R. C., Carr, S. J., Solomon, R. A., O'Connor, M. E., et al. (1991). Three psychological treatments for bulimia nervosa: A comparative trial. *Archives of General Psychiatry, 48*, 463–469.

Falloon, I. R., Boy, J. L., McGill, C. W., Williamson, M., Razani, J., Moss, H. B., et al. (1985). Family management in the prevention of morbidity of schizophrenia: Clinical outcome of a two-year longitudinal study. *Archives of General Psychiatry, 42*, 887–896.

Fanselow, M. S. (1994). Neural organization of the defensive behavior system responsible for fear. *Psychonomic Bulletin and Review, 1*, 429–438.

Fanselow, M. S., & Kim, J. J. (1994). Acquisition of contextual Pavlovian fear conditioning is blocked by application of an NMDA receptor antagonist D, L-2-amino-5-phosphonovaleric acid to the basolateral amygdala. *Behavioral Neuroscience, 108*, 210–212.

Fanselow, M. S., & LeDoux, J. E. (1999). Why do we think plasticity underlying Pavlovian fear conditioning occurs in the basolateral amygdala? *Neuron, 23*, 229–232.

Fava, G. A., Bartolucci, G., Rafanelli, C., & Mangelli, L. (2001). Cognitive-behavioral management of patients with bipolar disorder who relapsed while on lithium prophylaxis. *Journal of Clinical Psychiatry, 62*, 556–559.

Fava, G. A., Grandi, S., Zielezny, M., Canestrari, R., & Morphy, M. A. (1994). Cognitive behavioral treatment of residual symptoms in primary major depressive disorder. *American Journal of Psychiatry, 151*, 1295–1299.

Fava, G. A., Grandi, S., Zielezny, M., Rafanelli, C., & Canestrari, R. (1996). Four-year outcome for cognitive behavioral treatment of residual symptoms in major depression. *American Journal of Psychiatry, 153*, 945–947.

Fava, G. A., Rafanelli, C., Grandi, S., Canestrari, R., and Morphy, M. A. (1998). Six-year outcome for cognitive behavioral treatment of residual symptoms in major depression. *American Journal of Psychiatry, 155*, 1443–1445.

Fava, G. A., Rafanelli, C., Grandi, S., Conti, S., & Belluardo, P. (1998). Prevention of recurrent depression with cognitive behavioral therapy: Preliminary findings. *Archives of General Psychiatry,* *55,* 816–820.

Fletcher, P. C., Happe, F., Frith, U., Baker, S. C., Dolan, R. J., Frackowiak, R. S. J., et al. (1995). Other minds in the brain: a functional imaging study of "theory of mind" in story comprehension. *Cognition, 57,* 109–128.

Fortin, N. J., Agster, K. L., & Eichenbaum, H. B. (2002). Critical role of the hippocampus in memory for sequences of events. *Nature Neurosciences, 5*(5), 458–462.

Foulks, E. F., & Pena, J. M. (1995). Ethnicity and psychotherapy: A component in the treatment of cocaine addiction in African Americans. *Psychiatric Clinics of North America, 18,* 607–620.

Fordl, T., Meisenzahl, E. M., Setzsche, T., Born, C., Groll, C., Jager, et al. (2000). Hippocampal changes in patients with a first episode of major depression. *American Journal of Psychiatry, 159,* 1112–1118.

Frank, E., Grochocinski, V. J., Spanier, C. A., Buysse, D. J., Cherry, C. R., Houck, et al. (2000). Interpersonal psychotherapy and antidepressant medication: Evaluation of a sequential treatment strategy in women with recurrent major depression. *Journal of Clinical Psychiatry, 61*(1), 51–57.

Frank, E., Hlastala, S., Ritenour, A., Houck, P., Tu, X. M., Monk, T. H., et al. (1997). Inducing lifestyle regularity in recovering bipolar patients: Results from the maintenance therapies in bipolar disorder protocol. *Biological Psychiatry, 41,* 1165–1173.

Frank, E., Karp, J. F., & Rush, A. J. (1993). Efficacy of treatments for major depression. *Psychopharmacology Bulletin, 29,* 457–475.

Frank, E., Kupfer, D. J., Gibbons, R., Houck, P., Kostelnik, B., Mallinger, et al. (in press). Interpersonal and social rhythm therapy prevents depressive symptomatology in patients with bipolar I disorder. *Archives of General Psychiatry.*

Frank, E., Kupfer, D. J., Perel, J. M., Cornes, C., Jarrett, D. B., Mallinger, A. G., et al. (1990). Three-year outcomes for maintenance therapies in recurrent depression. *Archives of General Psychiatry, 47,* 1093–1099.

Frank, E., Kupfer, D. J., Wagner, E. F., McEachran, A. B., & Cornes, C. (1991). Efficacy of interpersonal psychotherapy as a maintenance treatment of recurrent depression: Contributing factors. *Archives of General Psychiatry, 48,* 1053–1059.

Frank, E., Swartz, H. A., & Kupfer, D. J. (2000). Interpersonal and social rhythm therapy: Managing the chaos of bipolar disorder. *Biological Psychiatry, 48*, 593–604.

Frank, E., Swartz, H. A., Mallinger, A. G., Thase, M. E., Weaver, E. V., & Kupfer, D. J. (1999). Adjunctive psychotherapy for bipolar disorder: Effects of changing treatment modality. *Journal of Abnormal Psychology, 108*, 579–587.

Fredrikson, M., Wik, G., Greitz, T., Eriksson, L., Stone-Elander, S., Ericson, K., & et al. (1993). Regional cerebral blood flow during experimental phobic fear. *Psychophysiology, 30*, 126–30.

Freeman, C. P. L., Barry, F., Dunkeld-Turnbull, J., & Henderson, A. (1988). Controlled trial of psychotherapy for bulimia nervosa. *British Medical Journal, 296*, 521–525.

Freud, S. (1964). A disturbance of memory on the Acropolis. In J. Strachey (Ed. & Trans.), *The standard edition of the complete psychological works of Sigmund Freud* (Vol. 22, pp. 239–248). London: Hogarth Press. (Original work published in 1936).

Freud, S. (1966a). Project for a scientific psychology. In J. Strachey (Ed. & Trans.), *The standard edition of the complete psychological works of Sigmund Freud* (Vol. 1, pp. 233–239). London: Hogarth Press. (Original work published in 1895)

Freud, S. (1966b). Stratification of memory traces (Letter 52). In J. Strachey (Ed. & Trans.), *The standard edition of the complete psychological works of Sigmund Freud* (Vol. 1, pp. 233–239). London: Hogarth Press. (Original work published in 1950).

Friedman, A. S. (1975). Interaction of drug therapy with marital therapy in depressed patients. *Archives of General Psychiatry, 32*, 619–637.

Frodl, T., Meisenzahl, E. Zetzsche, T., Bottlender, R., Born, C., Groll, C., et al. (2002). Enlargement of the amygdala in patients with a fist episode of major depression. *Biological Psychiatry, 51*, 708–714.

Fromm-Reichmann, F. (1947). Problems of therapeutic management in a psychoanalytic hospital. *Psychoanalytic Quarterly, 16*, 325–356.

Furmark, T., Tillfors, M., Marteinsdottir, I., Fischer, H., Pissiota, A., Langstrom, B., et al. (2002). Common changes in cerebral blood flow in patients with social phobia treated with citalopram or cognitive-behavioral therapy. *Archives of General Psychiatry, 59,* 425–433.

Gabbard, G. O. (2000). A neurobiologically informed perspective on psychotherapy. *British Journal of Psychiatry, 177,* 117–122.

George, M. S., & Ketter, T. A. (1997). Depressed subjects have decreased rCBF activation during facial emotion recognition. *CNS Spectrums, 2*(10), 45–55.

Geschwind, D. N. (2000). Mice, microarrays, and the genetic diversity of the brain. *PNAS, 97,* 1076–1078.

Goldberg, R. S., Riba, M., & Tasman, A. (1991). Psychiatrists' attitudes toward prescribing medication for patients treated by non-medical psychotherapists. *Hospital and Community Psychiatry, 42,* 276–280.

Goldman, W., McCulloch, J., Cuffel, B., Zarin, D. A., Suarez, A., & Burns, B. J. (1998). Outpatient utilization patterns of integrated and split psychotherapy and pharmacotherapy for depression. *Psychiatric Services, 49,* 477–482.

Goldsmith, R. J., Paris, M., & Riba, M. B. (1999). Negative aspects of collaborative treatment. In M. B. Riba & R. Balon (Eds.), *Psychopharmacology and psychotherapy: A collaborative approach* (pp. 33–63). Washington, DC: American Psychiatric Press.

Gorman, J. M., Kent, J. M., Sullivan, G. M., & Coplan, J. D. (2000). Neuroanatomical hypothesis of panic disorder, revised. *American Journal of Psychiatry, 157,* 493–506.

Gottschalk, L. A. (1999). The application of a computerized measurement of the content analysis of natural language to the assessment of the effects of psychoactive drugs. *Methods and Findings in the Experimental and Clinical Pharmacology, 21,* 133–138.

Gottschalk, L. A. (2002). *Psychoanalysis and computerized content analysis of natural language and the measurement of neurobiological dimensions.* Unpublished manuscript.

Gottschalk, L. A., Buchsbaum, M. S., Gillin, J. C., Wu, J., Reynolds, C., & Herrera, D. B. (1991). Positron-emission tomographic studies of the relationship of cerebral glucose metabolism and the magnitude of anxiety and hostility experienced during dreaming and waking. *The Journal of Neuropsychiatry and Clinical Neurosciences, 3,* 131–142.

Gould, E., Beylin, A., Tanapat, P., Reeves, A., & Shors, T. J. (1999). Learning enhances adult neurogenesis in the hippocampal formation. *Nature Neuroscience, 2,* 260–265.

Gregory, R. J., & Jindal, R. D. (2001). Ethical dilemmas in prescribing antidepressants. *Archives of General Psychiatry, 58,* 1085–1086.

Griest, J. H., Jefferson, J. W., Kobak, K. A., Katzelnick, D. J., & Serlin, R. C. (1995). Efficacy and tolerability of serotonin transport inhibitors in obsessive-compulsive disorder. *Archives of General Psychiatry, 52,* 53–60.

Grigsby, J., & Stevens, D. (2002). Memory, neurodynamics, and human relationships. *Psychiatry, 65*(1), 13–34.

Grinspoon, L., Ewalt, J. R., & Shader, R. I. (1972). *Schizophrenia: Pharmacotherapy and psychotherapy.* Baltimore: Williams & Wilkins.

Hafner, J., & Marks, I. (1976). Exposure in vivo of agoraphobics: Contributions of diazepam, group exposure, and anxiety evocation. *Psychological Medicine, 6,* 71–88.

Hagman, J. Buchsbaum, M., Wu, J. C., Rao, S. J., Reynolds, C. A., & Blinder, B. J. (1990). Comparison of regional brain metabolism in bulimia nervosa and affective disorder assessed with positron emission tomography. *Journal of Affective Disorders, 19,* 153–162.

Hall, R. C. W., Beresford, R. R., Blow, F. C., & Hall, A. K. (1990). Differing physical from psychiatric disorders. In M .E. Thase, B. A. Edelstein, & M. Hersen (Eds.) *Handbook of outpatient treatment of adults: Nonpsychotic mental disorders* (pp. 19–40). New York: Plenum Press.

Hamilton, M. (1960). A rating scale for depression. *Journal of Neurology, Neurosurgery, and Psychiatry, 23,* 56–62.

Hansen-Grant, S., & Riba, M. (1995). Contact between psychotherapists and psychiatric residents who provide medication back up. *Psychiatric Services, 46,* 774–777.

Hersen, M., Bellack, A. S., Himmelhoch, J. M., & Thase, M. E. (1984). Effects of social skill training, amitriptyline, and psychotherapy in unipolar depressed women. *The Behavior Therapist, 15,* 21–40.

Herz, M. I., Endicott, J., Spitzer, R. L. (1977). Brief hospitalizations: A two-year follow-up. *American Journal of Psychiatry, 134,* 502–507.

Higgins, S. T., Delaney, D. D., Budney, A. J., Bickel, W. J., Hughes, J. R., Foerg, F., et al. (1991). A behavior approach to achieving initial cocaine abstinence. *American Journal of Psychiatry, 148,* 1218–1224.

Hlastala, S. A., Frank, E., Mallinger, A. G., Thase, M. E., Ritenour, A. M., & Kupfer, D. J. (1997). Bipolar depression: An underestimated treatment challenge. *Depression and Anxiety, 5,* 73–83.

Hogarty, G. E., Anderson, C. M., Reiss, D. J., Kornblith, S. J., Greenwald, D. P., Javna, C. D., et al. (1986). Family psychoeducation, social skills training, and maintenance chemotherapy in the aftercare treatment of schizophrenia. *Archives of General Psychiatry, 43,* 633–642.

Hogarty, G. E., Greenwald, D., Ulrich, R. F., Kornblith, S. J., DiBarry, A. L., Cooley, S., et al. (1997). Three-year trials of personal therapy among schizophrenic patients living with or independent of family, II: Effects on adjustment of patients. *American Journal of Psychiatry, 154,* 1514–1524.

Hogarty, G. E., Ulrich, R. F., Mussare, F., & Aristigueta, N. (1976). Drug discontinuation among long term, successfully maintained schizophrenic outpatients. *Diseases of the Nervous System, 37,* 494–500.

Hollon, S. D., DeRubeis, R. J., Evans, M. D., Wiemer, M. J., Garvey, M. J., Grove, W. M., et al. (1992). Cognitive therapy and pharmacotherapy for depression singly and in combination. *Archives of General Psychiatry, 49,* 774–781.

Horgan, C. M. (1985). Specialty and general ambulatory mental health services: Comparison of utilization and expenditures. *Archives of General Psychiatry, 42,* 565–572.

Hrobjartsson, A., & Gotzsche, P. C. (2001). Is the placebo powerless? An analysis of clinical trails comparing placebo with no treatment. *The New England Journal of Medicine, 344,* 1594–1602.

Huxley, N. A., Parikh, S. V., & Baldessarini, R. J. (2000). Effectiveness of psychosocial treatments in bipolar disorder: State of the evidence. *Harvard Review of Psychiatry, 8,* 126–140.

Jacobson, N. S., Dobson, K. S., Truax, P. A., Addis, M. E., Koerner, K., Gollan, J. K., et al. (1996). A component analysis of cognitive-behavioral treatment for depression. *Journal of Consulting and Clinical Psychology, 64,* 295–304.

Jamison, K. R. (1993). *Touched with fire: Manic depressive illness and the artistic temperament.* New York: Free Press.

Johnson, S. L., & Roberts, J. E. (1995). Life events and bipolar disorder: Implications from biological theories. *Psychological Bulletin, 117,* 434–449.

Johnson, S. L., Winett, C. A., Meyer, B., Greenhouse, W. J., & Miller, I. (1999). Social support and the course of bipolar disorder. *Journal of Abnormal Psychology, 108,* 558–566.

Joseph, R. (1996). *Neuropsychiatry, neuropsychology and clinical neuroscience.* Baltimore: Williams & Wilkins.

Kagan, J. (1995). *Galen's prophecy.* New York: Basic Books.

Kalin, N. H., Shelton, S. E., & Lynn, D. E. (1995). Opiate systems in mother and infant primates coordinate intimate contact during reunion. *Psychoneuroendocrinology,* 20(7), 735–742.

Kandel, E. R. (1998). A new intellectual framework for psychiatry. *American Journal of Psychiatry,* 155(4), 457–469.

Kandel, E. R. (1999a). Biology and the future of psychoanalysis: A new intellectual framework for psychiatry revisited. *American Journal of Psychiatry,* 156, 505–524.

Kandel, E. R. (1999b). Letter to editor. *American Journal of Psychiatry, 156,* 665–666.

Karasu, T. B. (1982). Psychotherapy and pharmacotherapy: Toward an integrative model. *American Journal of Psychiatry, 139,* 1102–1113.

Kay J. Integrated treatment: An overview. In J. Kay (Ed.), *Integrated treatment of psychiatric disorders* (pp. 1–29). Washington DC: American Psychiatric Press.

Keitner, G. I., & Miller, I. W. (1990). Family functioning and major depression: An overview. *American Journal of Psychiatry, 147,* 1128–1137.

Keitner, G. I., Ryan, C. E., Miller, W., Kohn, R., Bishop, D. S., & Epstein, N. B. (1995). Role of the family in recovery and major depression. *American Journal of Psychiatry, 152,* 1002–1008.

Keller, M. B., & Boland, R. J. (1998). Implications of failing to achieve successful long-term maintenance treatment of recurrent unipolar major depression. *Biological Psychiatry, 44,* 348–360.

Keller, M. B., McCullough, J. P., Klein, D. N., Arnow, B., Dunner, D. L., Gelenberg, A. J., et al. (2000). A comparison of nefazodone, the cognitive behavioral-analysis system of psychotherapy, and their combination for the treatment of chronic depression. *The New England Journal of Medicine, 342,* 1462–1470.

Kelly, K. V. (1992). Parallel treatment: Therapy with one clinician and medication with another. *Hospital and Community Psychiatry, 43,* 778–780.

Kemp, R., Kirov, G., Everitt, B., Hayard, P., & David, A. (1998). Randomized controlled trial of compliance therapy. *British Journal of Psychiatry, 172,* 413–419.

Kerber, K. B. (1999). Collaborative treatment in managed care. In M. B. Riba & R. Balon (Eds.), *Psychopharmacology and psychotherapy: A collaborative approach* (pp. 307–324). Washington, DC: American Psychiatric Press.

Khan, A., Warner, H. A., & Brown, W. A. (2000). Symptom reduction and suicide risk in patients treated with placebo in antidepressant clinical trials: An analysis of the Food and Drug Administration database. *Archives of General Psychiatry, 57,* 311–317.

Klein, E., Blinder, B. J., & Wu, J. (1996, May). *Caudate hypermetabolism in PET study of bulimia nervosa.* Paper presented to Society for Biological Psychiatry, New York, NY.

Klerman, G. L. (1991). Ideological conflicts in integrating pharmacotherapy and psychotherapy. In B. D. Beitman & G. L. Klerman (Eds.), *Integrating pharmacotherapy and psychotherapy* (pp. 3–20). Washington, DC: American Psychiatric Press.

Klerman, G. L., DiMascio, A., Weissman, M., Prusoff, B., & Paykel, E. (1974). Treatment of depression by drugs and psychotherapy. *American Journal of Psychiatry, 131,* 186–191.

Klerman, G. L., Weissman, M. M., Markowitz, J., Glick, I., Wilner, P. J., Mason, B., & Shear, M. K. (1994). Medication and psychotherapy. In A. E. Bergin & S. L. Garfield (Eds.), *Handbook of psychotherapy and behavior change* (pp. 734–782). New York: Raven.

Kluver, H., & Bucy, P. C. (1937). "Psychic blindness" and other symptoms following bilateral temporal lobe lobectomy in rhesus monkeys. *American Journal of Physiology, 119,* 352–353.

Kraemer, H. C., & Thiemann, S. (1987). *How many subjects? Statistical power analysis in research.* Newbury Park, CA: Sage Publications.

Kramer, P. D. (1992). *Listening to Prozac: A psychiatrist explores anti-depressant drugs and the remaking of the self.* New York: Viking.

Krupnick, J. L., Sotsky, S. M., Simmens, S., Moyer, J., E Watkins, J., et al. (1996). The role of therapeutic alliance chotherapy and pharmacotherapy outcome: Findings in the National Institute of Mental Health Treatment of Depression Collaborative Research Program. *Journal of Consulting and Clinical Psychology, 64*, 532–539.

Kuipers, E., Garety, P., Fowler, D., Dunn, G., Bebbington, P., Freeman, D., et al. (1997). London-East Anglia randomised controlled trial of cognitive-behavioural therapy psychosis. *British Journal of Psychiatry, 171*, 319–327.

Lam, D. H., Bright, J., Jones, S., Hayward, P., Schuck, N., Chisholm, D., et al. (2000). Cognitive therapy for bipolar illness—A pilot study of relapse prevention. *Cognitive Therapy and Research, 24*, 503–520.

Langs, R. (1973). *Psychoanalytical psychotherapy*, Vol. 1. New York: Jason Aronson.

Lauriello, J., Bustillo, J., & Keith, S. J. (1999). A criticial review of research on psychosocial treatment of schizophrenia. *Biological Psychiatry, 46*, 1409–1417.

Lavenex, P., & Amaral, D. G. (2000). Hippocampal-neocortical interaction: A hierarchy of associativity. *Hippocampus, 10*(4), 420–430.

Lavori, P. W. (1992). Clinical trials in psychiatry: Should protocol deviation censor patient data? *Neuropsychopharmacology, 6*, 39–48.

Lazarus, J. (1999). Ethical issues in collaborative or divided treatment. In M. B. Riba & R. Balon (Eds.), *Psychopharmacology and psychotherapy: A collaborative approach* (pp. 159–177). Washington, DC: American Psychiatric Press.

LeDoux, J. (2002). *Synaptic self: How our brain became who we are.* New York: Viking.

Leibenluft, E., Gardner, D. I., & Cowdrey, R. W. (1987). The inner experience of the borderline self-mutilator. *Journal of Personality Disorders, 1*, 317–324.

Levitt, J. J., McCarley, R. W., Dickey, C. C., & Voglmaier, M. M. (2002). MRI study of caudate nucleus volume and its cognitive correlates in neuroleptic-naïve patients with schizotypal personality disorder. *American Journal of Psychiatry, 159*, 1190–1197.

Liberman, R. P., Blackwell, G., Wallace, C. J., Mintz, J. (1994, May). Reducing relapse and rehospitalization in schizophrenic patients treated in a day hospital: A controlled study of skills training vs psychosocial occupational therapy. Presented at the 147th Annual Meeting of the American Psychiatric Association, Philadelphia, PA.

Liberman, R. P., Wallace, C. J., Blackwell, G., Kopelowicz, A., Vaccaro, J. V., & Mintz, J. (1998). Skills training versus psychosocial occupational therapy for persons with persistent schizophrenia. *American Journal of Psychiatry*, *155*, 1087–1091.

Luscher, C., Micoll, R., & Malenka, R. (2000). Synaptic plasticity and dynamic modulation of the posetsynaptic membrane. *Nature Neuroscience*, 3, 545–550

MacBeth, J. E. (1999). Divided treatment: Legal implications and risks. In M. B. Riba & R. Balon (Eds.), *Psychopharmacology and psychotherapy: A collaborative approach* (pp. 111–158). Washington, DC: American Psychiatric Press.

Main, T. F. (1957). The ailment. *British Journal of Medical Psychology*, *30*, 129–145.

Malenka, R. C. (2002). Synaptic Plasticity. In K. Davis, D. Charney, J. Coyle, C. Nermaroff (Eds.), *Neuropsychopharmacology: Fifth Generation of Progress*. Philadelphia: Lippincott Williams & Wilkins.

Manev, R., Uz, T., & Manev, H. (2001). Fluoxitene increases the content of neurotrophic protein S100B in the rat hippocampus. *European Journal of Pharmacology*, *420*, R1-R2.

Manev, H., Uz, T., Smalheiser, N. R., & Manev, R. (2001). Antidepressants alter cell proliferation on the adult brain in vivo and in neural cultures in vitro. *European Journal of Pharmacology*, *411*, 67–70.

Marder, S. R. Wirshing, W. C., Mintz, J., McKenzie, J., Johnston, K., Eckman, T. A., Lebell, M., Zimmerman, K., & Liberman, R. P. (1996). Two-year outcome of social skills training and group psychotherapy for outpatients with schizophrenia. *American Journal of Psychiatry*, *153*, 1585–1595.

Marks, I. M., Stern, R. S., Mawson, D., Cobb, J., & McDonald, R. (1980). Clomipramine and exposure for obsessive-compulsive rituals: I. *British Journal of Psychiatry*, *136*, 1–25.

Marks, I. M., Swinson, R. P., Basoglu, M., Kuch, K., Noshirvani, H., O'Sullivan, G., Lelliott, P. T., Kirby, M., McNamee, G., Sengun,

S., & Wickwire, K. (1993). Alprazolam and exposure alone and combined in panic disorder with agoraphobia: A controlled study in London and Toronto. *British Journal of Psychiatry, 162*, 776–787.

Martin, S. D., & Martin, E. (2001). Brain blood flow changes in depressed patients treated with interpersonal psychotherapy or Venlafaxine Hydrochloride. *Archives of General Psychiatry, 58*, 641–648.

Mavissakalian, M. R. (1995). Combined behavioral and pharmacological treatment of anxiety disorders. In L. J. Dickstein, M. B. Riba, & J. M. Oldham (Eds.), *Review of psychiatry*, (Vol. 15, pp. 565–584). Washington, DC: American Psychiatric Press.

Mawson, D., Marks, I. M., & Ramm, L. (1982). Clomipramine and exposure for chronic obsessive-compulsive rituals: III. Two year follow-up and further findings. *British Journal of Psychiatry, 140*, 11–18.

May, P. R. A. (1968). *Treatment of schizophrenia*. New York: Science House.

McConnaughy, E. A., DiClemente, C. C., Proschaska, J. O., & Velicer, W. F. (1989). Stage of change in psychotherapy: A follow-up report. *Psychotherapy, 26*, 494–503.

McCullough, J. P., Jr. (2000). *Treatment for chronic depression: Cognitive behavioral analysis system of psychotherapy*. New York: Guilford.

McKnight, D. L., Nelson-Gray, R. O., & Barnhill, J. (1992). Dexamethasone suppression test and response to cognitive therapy and antidepressant medication. *Behavior Therapist, 23*, 99–111.

Mesulam, M. M. (1981). A cortical network for directed attention and unilateral neglect. *Annals Neurology, 10*, 309–325.

Michaels, K. B. (2000). The placebo problem remains. *Archives of General Psychiatry, 57*, 321–322.

Miklowitz, D. J. (1998). Psychosocial approaches to the course and treatment of bipolar disorder. *CNS Spectrums, 3*, 48–52.

Miklowitz, D. J., Simoneau, T. L., George, E. L., Richards, J. A., Kalbag, A., Sachs-Ericsson, N., & Suddath, R. (2000). Family-focused treatment of bipolar disorder: 1-Year effects of a psychoeducational program in conjunction with pharmacotherapy. *Biological Psychiatry, 48*, 582–592.

Miller, I. W., & Keitner, G. I. (1996). Combined medication and psychotherapy in the treatment of chronic mood disorders. *Psychiatric Clinics of North America, 19,* 151–171.

Miller, I. W., Norman, W. H., & Keitner, G. I. (1989). Cognitive-behavioral treatment of depressed inpatients: Six- and twelve-month follow-up. *American Journal of Psychiatry, 146,* 1274–1279.

Miller, I. W., Norman, W. H., & Keitner, G. I. (1990). Treatment response of high cognitive dysfunction depressed inpatients. *Comprehensive Psychiatry, 30,* 62–71.

Mintz, D. (in press). Meaning and medication in the care of treatment resistant patients. *American Journal of Psychotherapy.*

Mischoulon, D., Rosenbaum, J. F., & Messner, E. (2000). Transfer to a new psychopharmacologist: Its effect on patients. *Academic Psychiatry, 24,* 156–163.

Mitchell, J. E., Pyle, R. L., Eckert, E. D., Hatasukami, D., Pomeroy, C., & Zimmerman, R. (1990). A comparison study of antidepressants and structured intensive group psychotherapy in the treatment of bulimia nervosa. *Archives of General Psychiatry, 47,* 149–157.

Mogg, K., & Bradley, B. P. (1999). Some methodological issues in assessing attentional biases for threatening faces in anxiety: A replication study using a modified version of the probe detection task. *Behavior Research & Therapy, 37*(6), 595–604.

Morisha, J. M. (Ed.) (2001). *Advances in Brain Imaging.* Washington: American Psychiatric Publishing.

Morris, J. S., Frith, C. D., Perret, D. I., Rowland, D., Young, A. W., Calder, A. J., & Dolan, R. J. (1996). A differential neural response in the human amygdala to fearful and happy facial expressions. *Nature, 383,* 812–815.

Morris, J. S., Ohman, A., & Dolan, R. J. (1998). Conscious and unconscious emotional learning in the human amygdala. *Nature, 393,* 467–470.

Morris, J. S., Ohman, A., & Dolan, R. J. (1999). A subcortical pathway to the right amygdala mediating "unseen" fear. *Proceedings of the National Academy Science USA, 96,* 1680–1685.

Murphy, G. E., Carney, R. M., Knesevich, M. A., Wetzel, R. D., & Whitworth, P. (1995). Cognitive behavior therapy, relaxation training, and tricyclic antidepressant medication in the treatment of depression. *Psychological Reports, 77,* 403–420.

Murphy, G. E., Simons, A. D., Wetzel, R. D., & Lustman, P. J. (1984). Cognitive therapy and pharmacotherapy. Singly and together in the treatment of depression. *Archives of General Psychiatry, 41,* 33–41.

Nadel, L., & Moskowitz, M. (1997). Memory consolidation retrograde amnesia and the hippocampal complex. *Current Opinion in Neurobiology, 7,* 217–227.

Nahm, F. K. D., Damasio, H., Tranel, D., & Damasio, A. (1993). Cross-modal associations and the human amygdala. *Neuropsychologia, 31,* 727–744.

Neal, D. L., & Calarco, M. M. (1999). Mental health providers: Role definitions and collaborative practice issues. In M. B. Riba & R. Balon (Eds.), *Psychopharmacology and psychotherapy: A collaborative approach* (pp. 85–109). Washington, DC: American Psychiatric Press.

Nesse, R. M. (2000). Is depression an adaptation? *Archives of General Psychiatry, 57,* 14–20.

O'Carroll, R. E., Drysdale, E., Cahill, L., Shajahan, P., & Ebmeier, K. P. (1999). Stimulation of the noradrenergic system enhances and blockade reduces memory for emotional material in man. *Psychological Medicine, 29*(5), 1083–1088.

O'Connor, K., Todorov, C., Robillard, S., Borgeat, F., & Brault, M. (1999). Cognitive-behaviour therapy and medication in the treatment of obsessive-compulsive disorder: A controlled study. *Canadian Journal of Psychiatry, 44,* 64–71.

Oldham, J. M. (2001). Integrated treatment planning for borderline personality disorder. In J. Kay (Ed.), *Integrated treatment of psychiatric disorders.* Washington, DC: American Psychiatric Publishing.

Olfson M., Marcus, S. C., Druss, B., Elinson, L., Tanielian, T., Pincus, H. A. (2002). National trends in the outpatient treatment of depression. *Journal of the American Medical Association, 287,* 203–209.

Otto, M. W., Pollack, M. H., Sachs, G. S., Reiter, S. R., Meltzer-Brody, S., & Rosenbaum, J. F. (1993). Discontinuation of benzodiazepine treatment: Efficacy of cognitive-behavioral therapy for patients with panic disorder. *American Journal of Psychiatry, 150,* 1485–1490.

Overall, J. E., & Gorham, D. E. (1961). The brief psychiatric rating scale. *Psychology Reports, 10,* 799–812.

Packard, M. G., & Cahill, L. (2001). Affective modulation of multiple memory systems. *Current Opinion Neurobiology, 11*(6), 752–756.

Pally, R. (1997a). How brain development is shaped by genetic and environmental factors. *International Journal of Psychoanalysis, 78*, 587–593.

Pally, R. (1997b). Memory: Brain systems that link past, present and future. *International Journal of Psychoanalysis, 78*, 1224–1234.

Pally, R. (1998a). Bilaterality: Hemispheric specialization and integration. *International Journal of Psychoanalysis, 79*, 565–578.

Pally, R. (1998b). Emotional processing: The mind body connection. *International Journal of Psychoanalysis, 79*, 349–362.

Pally, R. (2001). *The mind-brain relationship*. New York: Other Press.

Pally, R., & Olds, D. (1998). Consciousness: A neuroscience perspective. *International Journal of Psychoanalysis, 79*, 971–989.

Palmer, A. G., Williams, H., & Adams, M. (1995). CBT in a group format for bi-polar affective disorder. *Behavioural and Cognitive Psychotherapy, 23*, 153–168.

Panksepp, J. (1998). *Affective neuroscience*. New York: Oxford University Press.

Paul, G. L., & Lentz, R. J. (1977). *Psychosocial treatment of chronic mental patients*. Cambridge, MA: Harvard University Press.

Paul, G. L., Tobias, L. L., & Holly, B. L. (1972). Maintenance psychotropic drugs in the presence of active treatment programs. *Archives of General Psychiatry, 27*, 106–115.

Paykel, E. S. (1995). Psychotherapy, medication combinations, and compliance. *Journal of Clinical Psychiatry, 56* (Suppl. 1), 24–30.

Paykel, E. S., Scott, J., Teasdale, J. D., Johnson, A. L., Garland, A., Moore, R., et al. (1999). Prevention of relapse in residual depression by cognitive therapy. *Archives of General Psychiatry, 56*, 829–835.

Penn, D., & Mueser, K. (1996). Research update on the psychosocial treatment of schizophrenia. *American Journal of Psychiatry, 153*, 607–617.

Perris, C. (1989). *Cognitive therapy of schizophrenia*. New York: Guilford.

Perry, A., Tarrier, N., Morriss, R., McCarthy, E., & Limb, K. (1999). Randomized controlled trial of efficacy of teaching patients with bipolar disorder to identify early symptoms of relapse and obtain treatment. *British Medical Journal, 318,* 149–153.

Phillips, R. G, & LeDoux, J. E. (1992). Differential contribution of amygdala and hippocampus to cued and contextual fear conditioning. *Behavioral Neurosci*ence, *106,* 274–285.

Pilette, W. L. (1988). The rise of three-party treatment relationships. *Psychotherapy, 25,* 420–423.

Pine, D. S. (2001). *Functional neuroimaging in children and adolescents in advances in brain imaging.* Washington, DC: American Psychiatric Press.

Prochaska, J. O., Norcross, J. C., & DiClemente, C. C. (1995). *Changing for good.* New York: Avon.

Project MATCH Research Group. (1997). Matching alcoholism treatment to client heterogeneity: Project MATCH post-treatment drinking outcomes. *Journal of the Study of Alcohol, 58,* 7–29.

Prusoff, B. A., Weissman, M. M., Klerman, G. L., & Rounsaville, B. J. (1980). Research diagnostic criteria subtypes of depression: Their role as predictors of differential response to psychotherapy and drug treatment. *Archives of General Psychiatry, 37,* 796–801.

Quartz, S. R., & Sejnowski, T. J. (1997). The neural basis of cognitive development: A constructivist manifesto. *Behavioral and Brain Sciences,* 20, 537–556.

Quitkin, F. M., Stewart, J. W., McGrath, P. J., Tricamo, E., Rabkin, J. G., Ocepek-Welikson, K., et al. (1993). Columbia atypical depression. A subgroup of depressives with better response to MAOI than to tricyclic antidepressants or placebo. *British Journal of Psychiatry, 163*(Suppl. 21), 30–34.

Randolph, E. T., Eth, S., Glynn, S. M., Paz, G. G., Leong, G. B., Shaner, A. L., et al. (1994). Behavioural family management in schizophrenia: Outcome of a clinic-based intervention. *British Journal of Psychiatry, 164,* 501–506.

Rappaport, D. (1942). *Emotions and memory.* New York: International University Press.

Rappaport, D. (1953). On the psychoanalytic theory of affects. *International Journal Psychoanalysis, 34,* 177–198.

Rappaport, D. (1967). *Collected papers.* New York: Basic Books.

Ravindran, A. V., Anisman, H., Merali, Z., Charbonneau, Y., Telner, J., Bialik, R. J., Weins, A., Ellis, J., & Griffiths, J. (1999). Treatment of primary dysthymia with group cognitive therapy and pharmacotherapy: Clinical symptoms and functional impairments. *American Journal of Psychiatry, 156,* 1608–1617.

Regier, D. A., Boyd, J. H., Burke, J. D., Jr., Rae, D. S., Myers, J. K., Kramer, M., Robins, L. N., George, L. K., Karno, M., & Locke, B. Z. (1988). One-month prevalence of mental disorders in the United States: Based on five epidemiological catchment area sites. *Archives of General Psychiatry, 45,* 977–986.

Regier, D. A., Goldberg, I. D., & Taube, C. A. (1978). The de facto U.S. mental health services system: A public health perspective. *Archives of General Psychiatry, 35,* 685–693.

Reynolds, C. F., III, Frank, E., Perel, J. M., Imber, S. D., Cornes, C., Miller, M. D., et al. (1999). Nortriptyline and interpersonal psychotherapy as maintenance therapies for recurrent major depression: A randomized controlled trial in patients older than 59 years. *Journal of the American Medical Association, 281,* 39–45.

Riba, M. B., Goldberg, R. S., & Tasman A. (1993). Medication backup in psychiatry residency programs. *Academic Psychiatry, 17,* 32–35.

Riba, M. B., & Tasman, A. (2000). Managing difficult cases. In A. Tasman, M. B. Riba, & K. R. Silk (Eds.), *The doctor-patient relationship in pharmacotherapy: Improving treatment effectiveness* (pp. 147–169). New York: Guilford.

Ribeiro, S. C. M., Tandon, R., Grunhaus, L., & Greden, J. F. (1993). The DST as a predictor of outcome in depression: A meta-analysis. *American Journal of Psychiatry, 150,* 1618–1629.

Rosenheck, R., Tekell, J., Peters, J., Cramer, J., Fontana, A., Xu, W., et al. (1998). Does participation in psychosocial treatment augment the benefit of clozapine? *Archives of General Psychiatry, 55,* 618–625.

Rounsaville, B. J., Klerman, G. L., & Weissman, M. M. (1981). Do psychotherapy and pharmacotherapy for depression conflict? Empirical evidence from a clinical trial. *Archives of General Psychiatry, 38,* 24–29.

Ruiz, P., Venegas-Samuels, K., & Alarcon, R. (1995). The economics of pain: Mental health care costs among minorities. *Psychiatric Clinics of North America, 18,* 659–670.

Sabo, A. N., & Rand, B. I. (2000). The relational aspects of psychopharmacology. In A. N. Sabo & L. Havens (Eds.), *The real world guide to psychotherapy practice* (pp. 34–62). Cambridge, MA: Harvard University Press.

Sachs, G. S., & Thase, M. E. (2000). Bipolar disorder therapeutics: Maintenance treatment. *Biological Psychiatry, 48*(6), 573–581.

Sackeim, H. A. (2001). Functional brain circuits in major depression and remission. *Archives of General Psychiatry, 58,* 649–650.

Schacter, D. L. (1992). Priming and multiple memory systems: Perceptual mechanisms of implicit memory. *Journal Cognitive Neuroscience, 4,* 244–256.

Schacter, D. L., Reiman, E., Curran, T., Yun, L. S., Bandy, D., McDermott, K. B., et al. (1996). Neuroanatomical correlates of veridical and illusory recognition memory: Evidence from positron emission tomography. *Neuron, 17,* 1–20.

Schacter, D. L. (2001). *The seven sins of memory.* Boston: Houghton Mifflin.

Shankle, W. R., Landing, B. R., Hara, J. & Fallon, J. (1998). Constructing the human cerebral cortex duing infancy and childhood: Types and numbers of cortical columns and numbers of neurons in such columns at different age points. *Acta Pediatrica Japanica, 40*(6): 530–543.

Schatzberg, A. F. (2002). Major depression: Causes or effects?. *American Journal of Psychiatry, 159,* 1077–1079.

Schooler, N. R. (1978). Antipsychotic drugs and psychological treatment in schizophrenia. In M. A. Lipton, A. DiMascio, & K. F. Killam (Eds.), *Psychopharmacology: A generation of progress* (pp. 1155–1168). New York: Raven.

Schooler, N. R., Keith, S. J., Severe, J. B., Matthews, S. M., Bellack, A. S., Glick, I. D., et al. (1997). Relapse and rehospitalization during maintenance treatment of schizophrenia: The effects of dose reduction and family treatment. *Archives of General Psychiatry, 54,* 453–463.

Schooler, N. R., Levine, J., Severe, J. B., Brauzer, B., DiMascio, A., Klerman, G. L., et al. (1980). Prevention of relapse in schizophrenia: An evaluation of fluphenazine decanoate. *Archives of General Psychiatry, 37,* 16–24.

Schore, A. N. (1994). *Affect Regulation and the Origin of the Self.* Hillsdale, NJ: Lawrence Erlbaum.

Schulberg, H. C., Block, M. R., Madonia, M. J., Scott, C. P., Rodriguez, E., Imber, S. D., et al. (1996). Treating major depression in primary care practice: Eight-month clinical outcomes. *Archives of General Psychiatry, 53,* 913–919.

Schwartz, J. M. (1996). *Brain lock.* New York: Regan Books.

Schwartz, J. M., Stoessel, P. W., Baxter, L. R., Martin, K. M., & Phelps, M. E. (1996). Systematic changes in cerebral glucose metabolic rate after successful behavior modification treatment of obsessive-compulsive disorder. *Archives of General Psychiatry, 53,* 109–113.

Sciolla, A. (2001, May 18). Psychotherapy training: The neurobiology behind the talk. *Psychiatric News, 36*(10), 13.

Scott, J. (1996). Cognitive therapy of affective disorders: A review. *Journal of Affective Disorders, 37,* 1–11.

Seligman, M. E. P. (1995). The effectiveness of psychotherapy. The Consumer Reports study. *American Psychologist, 50,* 965–974.

Shankle, W. R., Landing, B. H., Hara, J., & Fallon, J. (1998). Constructing the human cerebral cortex during infancy and childhood: Types and numbers of cortical columns and numbers of neurons in such columns at different age-points. *Acta Paediatrica Japonica, 40*(6), 530–543.

Sherbourne, C. D., Hays, R. D., Ordway, L., DiMatteo M. R., & Kravitz, R. L. (1992). Antecedents of adherence to medical recommendations: Results from medical outcomes study. *Journal of Behavioral Medicine, 15,* 447–468.

Shors, T. J., Miesegaes, G., Beylin, A., Zhao, M., Rydel, T., & Gould, E. (2001). Neurogenesis in the adult is involved in the formation of trace memories. *Nature, 410,* 314–315, 317.

Siegel, D. J. (1996). Cognition, memory, and dissociation. *Child and Adolescent Psychiatric Clinics of North America, 5,* 509–536.

Silk, K. R. (1999). Collaborative treatment for patients with personality disorders. In M. B. Riba & R. Balon (Eds.), *Psychopharmacology and psychotherapy: A collaborative approach* (pp. 221–277). Washington, DC: American Psychiatric Press.

Silk, K. R., Lee, S., & Hill, E. M. (1995). Borderline symptoms and severity of sexual abuse. *American Journal of Psychiatry, 152,* 1059–1064.

Smith, J. M. (1989). Some dimensions of transference in combined treatment. In J. M. Ellison (Ed.), *The psychotherapist's guide to pharmacotherapy* (pp. 79–94). Chicago: Year Book Medical.

Smith, M. T., Perlis, M. L., Park, A., Smith, M. S. Pennington, J., Giles, D. E., & Buysse, D. J. (2002). Comparative meta-analysis of pharmacotherapy and behavior therapy for persistent insomnia. American Journal of Psychiatry, *159*, 5–11.

Spanier, C., Frank, E., McEachran, A. B., Grochocinski, V. J., & Kupfer, D. J. (1996). The prophylaxis of depressive episodes in recurrent depression following discontinuation of drug therapy: Integrating psychological and biological factors. *Psychological Medicine, 26*, 461–475.

Spiegel, D. A., & Bruce, T. J. (1997). Benzodiazepines and exposure-based cognitive behavior therapies for panic disorder: Conclusion from combined treatment trials. *American Journal of Psychiatry, 154*, 773–781.

Spiegel, D. A., Bruce, T. J., Gregg, S. F., & Nuzzarello, A. (1994). Does cognitive behavior therapy assist in slow-taper alprazolam discontinuation in panic disorder? *American Journal of Psychiatry, 151*, 876–881.

Spitz, D., Hansen-Grant, S., & Riba, M. B. (1999). Residency training issues in collaborative treatment. In M. B. Riba & R. Balon (Eds.), *Psychopharmacology and psychotherapy: A collaborative approach* (pp. 325–352). Washington, DC: American Psychiatric Press.

Spitzer, R. L., Endicott, J., & Robins, E. (1978). Research diagnostic criteria: Rationale and reliability. *Archives of General Psychiatry, 35*, 773–782.

Springer, T., Huth, A. C., Lohr, N. E., & Silk, K. R. (1995, August*). The quality of depression in personality disorders: An empirical study*. Paper presented at the annual meeting of the American Psychological Association, New York, NY.

Stewart, J. W., Garfinkel, R., Nunes, E. V., Donovan, S., & Klein, D. F. (1998). Atypical features and treatment response in the National Institute of Mental Health Treatment of Depression Collaborative Research Program. *Journal of Clinical Psychopharmacology, 18*, 429–434.

Stewart, J. W., Mercier, M. A., Agosti, V., Guardino, M., & Quitkin, F. M. (1993). Imipramine is effective after unsuccessful cognitive therapy: Sequential use of cognitive therapy and imipramine in depressed outpatients. *Journal of Clinical Psychopharmacology, 13,* 114–119.

Tasman, A, & Riba, M. B. (2000). Psychological management in psychopharmacologic treatment. In J. Lieberman & A. Tasman (Eds.), *Psychiatric drugs* (pp. 242–249). Philadelphia: W. B. Saunders.

Teasdale, J. D., Fennell, M. J. V., Hibbert, G. A., & Amies, P. L. (1984). Cognitive therapy for major depressive disorder in primary care. *British Journal of Psychiatry, 144,* 400–406.

Thase, M. E. (2000a). Psychopharmacology in conjunction with psychotherapy. In R. Ingram & R. C. Snyder (Eds.), *Handbook of psychological change: Psychotherapy process and practices for the 21st century* (pp. 474–497). New York: Wiley.

Thase, M. (2001). Neuroimaging profiles and the differential therapies of depression. *Archives of General Psychiatry, 58,* 651–653.

Thase, M. E. (1996). The role of Axis II comorbidity in the management of patients with treatment resistant depression. *Psychiatric Clinics of North America, 19,* 287–309.

Thase, M. E. (1997). Integrating psychotherapy and pharmacotherapy for treatment of major depressive disorder: Current status and future considerations. *The Journal of Psychotherapy Practice and Research, 6,* 300–306.

Thase, M. E. (1999). How should efficacy be evaluated in randomized clinical trials of treatments for depression? *Journal of Clinical Psychiatry, 60*(Suppl. 4), 23–31.

Thase, M. E. (2000b). Recent developments in the pharmacotherapy of depression. *Psychiatric Clinics of North America: Annual of Drug Therapy, 7,* 151–171.

Thase, M. E. (2002). Studying new antidepressants: If there was a light at the end of the tunnel could we see it? *Journal of Clinical Psychiatry, 63*(Suppl. 2), 24–28.

Thase, M. E., Buysse, D. J., Frank, E., Cherry, C. R., Cornes, C. L., Mallinger, A. G., et al. (1997). Which depressed patients will respond to interpersonal psychotherapy? The role of abnormal electroencephalographic sleep profiles. *American Journal of Psychiatry, 154,* 502–509.

Thase, M. E., Dubé, S., Bowler, K., Howland, R. H., Myers, J. E., Friedman, E., et al. (1996). Hypothalamic-pituitary-adrenocortical activity and response to cognitive behavior therapy in unmedicated, hospitalized depressed patients. *American Journal of Psychiatry, 153*, 886–891.

Thase, M. E., Entsuah, A. R., & Rudolph, R. L. (2001). Remission rates during treatment with venlafaxine or selective serotonin reuptake inhibitors. *British Journal of Psychiatry, 178*, 234–241.

Thase, M. E., Fasiczka, A. L., Berman, S. R., Simons, A. D., & Reynolds, C. F., III. (1998). Electroencephalographic sleep profiles before and after cognitive behavior therapy of depression. *Archives of General Psychiatry, 55*, 138–144.

Thase, M. E., Fava, M., Halbreich, U., Kocsis, J. H., & Koran, L. (1996). A placebo-controlled randomized clinical trial comparing sertraline and imipramine for the treatment of dysthymia. *Archives of General Psychiatry, 53*, 777–784.

Thase, M. E., Frank, E., Kornstein, S., & Yonkers, K. A. (2000). Gender differences in response to treatments of depression. In E. Frank (Ed.), *Gender and its effects on psychopathology* (pp. 103–129). Washington, DC: American Psychiatric Press.

Thase, M. E., & Friedman, E. S. (1999). Is psychotherapy, alone, an effective treatment for melancholia and other severe depressive states? *Journal of Affective Disorders, 54*, 1–19.

Thase, M. E., Greenhouse, J. B., Frank, E., Reynolds, C. F., III, Pilkonis, P. A., Hurley, K., et al. (1997). Treatment of major depression with psychotherapy or psychotherapy-pharmacotherapy combinations. *Archives of General Psychiatry, 54*, 1009–1015.

Thase, M. E., Kupfer, D. J., Fasiczka, A. L., Buysse, D. J., Simons, A. D., & Frank, E. (1997). Identifying an abnormal electroencephalographic sleep profile to characterize major depressive disorder. *Biological Psychiatry, 41*, 964–973.

Thase, M. E., Rush, A. J., Manber, R., Kornstien, S. G., Kliein, D. N. Markowtiz, J. C., et al. (2002). Differential effects of nefazodone and Cognitive Behavioral Analysis System of Psychotherapy on insomnia associated with chronic forms of depression. *Journal of Clinical Psychiatry, 63*, 493–500.

Thase, M. E., Simons, A. D., & Reynolds, C. F., III. (1996). Abnormal electroencephalographic sleep profiles in major depression. *Archives of General Psychiatry, 53*, 99–108.

Tran, P. V., Hamilton, S. H., Kuntz, A. J., Potvin, J. H., Andersen, S. W., Beasley, Jr. C., et al. (1997). Double-blind comparison of olanzapine versus risperidone in the treatment of schizophrenia and other psychotic disorders. *Journal of Clinical Psychopharmacology, 17,* 407–418.

Tranel, D., & Hyman, B. T. (1990). Neuropsychological correlates of bilateral amygdala damage. *Archives of Neurology, 47,* 349–355.

Valenstein, M. (1999). Primary care physicians and mental health professionals: Models for collaboration. In M. B. Riba & R. Balon (Eds.), *Psychopharmacology and psychotherapy: A collaborative approach* (pp. 325–352). Washington, DC: American Psychiatric Press.

van Balkom, A. J. L. M., De Haan, E., Van Oppen, P., Spinhoven, Hoogduin, K. A. L., & Van Dyck, R. (1998). Cognitive and behavioral therapies alone versus in combination with fluvoxamine in the treatment of obsessive-compulsive disorder. *The Journal of Nervous and Mental Disease, 186,* 492–499.

Van Praag, H., Schinder, A. F., Christie, B. R., Toni, N., Palmer, T. D., & Gage, F. H. (2002). Functional neurogenesis in the adult hippocampus. *Nature, 415*(6875), 1030–1034.

Varga-Kahdovan, F. (1997). Differential effects of early hippocampal pathology on episodic and semantic memory. *Science, 227,* 374–380.

Vaughn, C. E., & Leff, J. P. (1976). The influence of family and social factors on the course of psychiatric illness: A comparison of schizophrenic and depressed neurotic patients. *British Journal of Psychiatry, 129,* 125–137.

Viinamak, H., Kuikka, J., Tiihonen, J., & Lehtonen, J. (1998). Change in monoamine transporter density related to clinical recovery: A case-control study. *Nordic Journal of Psychiatry, 52,* 39–44.

Wall, P. M., & Messier, C. (2001). The hippocampal formation—orbitomedial prefrontal cortex circuit in the attentional control of active memory. *Behavioral Brain Research, 127*(1–2), 99–117.

Walsh, B. T., & Devlin, M. J. (1995). Psychopharmacology of anorexia nervosa, bulimia nervosa, and binge eating. In F. E. Bloom & D. J. Kupfer (Eds.), *Psychopharmacology: The fourth generation of progress* (pp. 1581–1589). New York: Raven.

Walsh, B. T., Wilson, G. T., Loeb, K. L., Devlin, M. J., Pike, K. M., Roose, S. P., et al. (1997). Medication and psychotherapy in the treatment of bulimia nervosa. *American Journal of Psychiatry, 154*, 523–531.

Ward, N. (1991). Psychosocial approaches to pharmacotherapy. In B. D. Beitman & G. L. Klerman (Eds.), *Integrating pharmacotherapy and psychotherapy*. Washington, DC: American Psychiatric Press.

Wardle, J. (1990). Behavior therapy and benzodiazepines: Allies or antagonists? *British Journal of Psychiatry, 156*, 163–168.

Weiner, H., & Riba, M. B. (1997). Attitudes and practices in medication backup. *Psychiatric Services, 48*, 536–538.

Wells, K. B., Burnam, M. A., Rogers, W., Hays, R., & Camp, R. (1992). The course of depression in adult outpatients: Results from the Medical Outcomes Study. *Archives of General Psychiatry, 49*, 788–794.

Weston, D., & Gabbard, G. O. (2002). Developments in Cognitive Neuroscience: II. Implications for theories of transference. *Journal of the American Psychoanalytic Association, 50*, 99–134.

Whalen, P. J., Rauch, S. L., Etcoff, N. L., McInerney, S. C., Lee, M. B., & Jenike, M. A. (1998). Masked presentations of emotional facial expressions modulate amygdala activity without explicit knowledge. *The Journal of Neuroscience, 18*, 411–418.

Whisman, M. A. (1993). Mediators and moderators of change in cognitive therapy of depression. *Psychological Bulletin, 114*, 248–265.

Wickeloren, I. (1997). Getting a grasp on working memory. *Science, 275*, 1580–1582.

Wik, G., Fredrikson, M., Ericson, K. Eriksson, L., Stone-Elander, S., & Grietz, T. (1993). A functional cerebral response to frightening visual stimulation. *Psychiatry Research, 50*, 15–24.

Wilson, M., Bell-Dolan, D., & Beitman, B. D. (1997). Application of stages of change scale in a clinical drug trial. *Journal of Anxiety Disorders, 10*, 331–345.

Woodward, B., Duckworth, K. S. & Gutheil, T. G. (1993). The pharmacotherapist-psychotherapist collaboration. In J. M. Oldham, M. B. Riba, & H. Tasman (Eds.), *Review of Psychiatry*, (Vol. 12, pp. 631–649). Washington, DC: American Psychiatric Press.

Woody, G. E., McLellan, A. T., & Luborsky, L. (1984). Psychiatric severity as a predictor of benefits from psychotherapy. *American Journal of Psychiatry, 141*, 1171–1177.

Woody, G. E., McLellan, A. T., Luborsky, L., O'Brien, C. P., Beck, A. T., Blaine, J., et al. (1983). Psychotherapy for opiate addicts: Does it help? *Archives of General Psychiatry, 40,* 639–645.

Wu, J. C., Hagman, J., Buchsbaun, M. S., Blinder, B. J., Derrfler, M., Tai, W. Y., et al. (1990). Greater left cerebral hemispheric metabolism in bulimia assessed by positron emission tomography. *American Journal of Psychiatry, 147,* 309–312.

Yamamoto, J., Silva, J. A., Justice, L. R. (1993). Cross-cultural psychotherapy. In A. C. Gaw (Ed.), *Culture, ethnicity, and mental illness* (pp. 101–124). Washington, DC: American Psychiatric Press.

Yeh, S. R., Fricke, R. A., & Edwards, D. H. (1969). The effect of social experience on serotonergic modulation of the escape circuit of the crayfish. *Science, 271,* 366–369.

Young, R. C., Biggs, J. T., Siegler, V. E., & Meyer, D. A. (1978). A rating scale for mania: Reliability, validity, and sensitivity. *British Journal of Psychiatry, 133,* 429–435.

Zaretsky, A. E., Segal, Z. V., & Gemar, M. (1999). Cognitive therapy for bipolar depression: A pilot study. *Canadian Journal of Psychiatry, 44,* 491–494.

Ziedonis, D., Krejci, J., & Atdjian, S. (2001). Integrated treatment of alcohol, tobacco and other drug addictions. In J. Kay (Ed.), *Integrated treatment of psychiatric disorders* (pp. 79–111). Washington, DC: American Psychiatric Publishing.

Zucker, R (1999). Calcium and activity-dependent synaptic plasticity. *Current Opinion in Neurobiology 9,* 305–313.

Zwillig, T. (1999). Anxiety builds over jump in liability for prescribing errors: Insurers pay more for prescribing error claims than for psychotherapy claims. *Clinical Psychiatry News, 27,* 1, 5.

Index

adherence (to medication regimen)
  assessment of nonadherence risk,
    37–40
  case vignettes, 43–45, 49–50, 51–53,
    58, 59–61, 63, 65–66, 67, 68, 96–97
  dietary restrictions and, 45, 63
  family factors in, 58–59, 71
  implications for psychotherapy, 15
  obstacles to, 37, 65, 117
  patient attitude toward authority and,
    26–27, 31
  patient rationalizations for
    discontinuation, 54, 55–56, 66, 70
  role of psychotherapy in promoting,
    37, 40–42, 43–45, 49–53, 54, 55, 58,
    59–62, 63, 70, 76–77, 117–118
  side effects and, 49, 50, 51–53, 54, 61,
    66, 76–77, 82
  split treatment and, 149
  therapeutic relationship and, 35–36
  in therapy termination, 36
  transference issues in, 45–46, 63
alprazolam, 127–128
amitriptyline, 95, 123
amygdala, 106, 165–171, 172, 173,
  175–176; *see also* neurobiology of
  psychotherapy
anorexia nervosa
  initiating pharmacotherapy, 43–44, 63
  neurobiology of, 176–177
anterior cingulate cortex, 173–174; *see
  also* neurobiology of psychotherapy

anxiety disorders, 4, 122
  neurobiological model, 105–106, 166,
    174–177
  treatment outcomes, 129–130
assessment
  indications for split treatment, 79,
    82–83
  panic disorder, 89–90
  risk of medication nonadherence,
    37–40
Ativan. *see* lorazepam
attachment processes, 176
attentional processes, 164–165

basal ganglia, 170; *see also* neurobiology
  of psychotherapy
behavior therapy, 5–6
benzodiazepines, 19–20, 31, 103, 130
  in combined therapy, 127–128
  panic disorder treatment, 6, 127–128
  withdrawal, 7
beta-blockers, 130
bipolar disorder, 24, 29–30, 75, 86
  case vignettes, 26, 41–42, 43, 63
  psychopharmacotherapy rationale, 4,
    11
  treatment outcomes, 136–138
borderline disorder, 57–58, 148, 154
  treatment matching, 88
  typology, 88
Brain Lock, 23
bulimia, 4, 122, 176

neurobiology of, 176–177
treatment effectiveness, 5–6, 130–131
buspirone, 130
butalbital, 20–21

carbamazepine, 120
caudate nucleus, 167, 176; *see also*
neurobiology of psychotherapy
ceiling effects, 113–114
change processes
additive effects in combined therapy,
113–117
initiating new patterns of behavior,
20–21, 32
neurobiology of psychotherapy, 105,
106–108, 161–162, 170–172, 175,
178–179
role of pharmacotherapy in, 15–16
substages of, initiation of
pharmacotherapy in, 22, 29
in supportive psychotherapy, 68
character and temperament, 88
circuits model, 105–106
clomipramine, 129
clonazepam, 26, 47, 64, 98, 99
clozapine, 135
cognitive behavior analysis system of
psychotherapy, 125
cognitive behavior therapy (CBT), 87
anxiety disorder treatment, 129–130
bipolar disorder treatment, 137
in combined therapy for depression,
123–125, 126–127
eating disorder treatment, 5–6,
130–131
panic disorder treatment, 6, 127–129
schizophrenia treatment, 133,
134–135
substance abuse treatment, 132
cognitive functioning
discrepancy detection, 164–165
hypervigilence, 177
neurobiology, 172–174
cognitive therapy (CT), 87, 89
depression treatment, 5
to promote medication adherence,
37–40
combined treatment
for anxiety disorders, 129–130
for bipolar disorder, 136–138
case vignettes, 16–31, 41–68
definition, *xvii*, 90
for depression, 123–127
for eating disorders, 130–131
effectiveness, 3, 5–6, 111–112,
118–119, 122, 138
indications, 122

for obsessive-compulsive disorder
(OCD), 129
for panic disorder, 127–129
psychotherapeutic significance of
pharmacotherapy practice, 13–16,
36, 80, 81, 83
research needs, 112, 138–139
role of psychotherapy in
pharmacotherapy, 35–41, 69,
144–145
for schizophrenia, 133–135
stages of treatment, 14–15
for substance abuse, 131–132
termination, 16, 36
termination of pharmacotherapy, 68
see also integrated treatment;
psychotherapy with
pharmacotherapy; sequencing of
therapies
compliance. *see* adherence
compliance therapy, 37, 38–40
confidentiality, 74, 151
couples therapy and, 77–78, 82
in split treatment, 156–157
constructivism, 171
contingency management, 135
countertransference, *xvii*
split treatment and, 151–152, 158
termination issues, 24–25, 30, 57, 67
couples therapy, 18, 28, 74, 77–78, 81, 83
culturally sensitive practice, 147–148

deficit matching, 86–87
Depakote. *see* divalproex sodium
depression, 4, 122
case vignettes, 46–49, 50, 52, 59,
62–63, 68, 69
combined therapy, 5, 115, 119,
123–127, 138
monotherapy, 4, 5
neurobiology, 175
pharmacotherapy, 46–47, 63
self-value issues in, 48–49, 64–65
treatment effectiveness, 115, 119
desipramine, 131, 132
Desyrel. *see* trazodone
diazepam, 127
disulfiram, 131, 132
divalproex sodium, 26, 120
dopaminergic system, 176; *see also*
neurobiology of psychotherapy
dreaming, 177–178
drug development and approval process,
119–120
duration of pharmacotherapy, 23, 29,
121
dysthymia, 4, 16–17

Effexor. *see* venlafaxine
emotional functioning, 165–171
    in dreams, 177–178
    neurobiological model of
        psychopathology, 174–177
ethical issues in split treatment, 153–156
exposure desensitization, 89, 127–128

family-focused therapy, 136–137
family therapy, 5, 134
fear response, 165–166, 177
Fiorinal. *see* butalbital
fluoxetine, 131
Food and Drug Administration, U.S.
    (FDA), 119–120

gabapentin, 51–52
gene transcription function, *xvi*
glucose metabolism, 166–167
grief reactions, 16, 31
    in loss of marriage, 22, 29, 32
    in termination of therapy, 32

hippocampus, 162–165, 166, 167, 169,
    172, 175; *see also* neurobiology of
    psychotherapy
hypothalamus, 166; *see also*
    neurobiology of psychotherapy

imipramine, 44, 51, 63, 126, 128, 130
insomnia, 4, 122
integrated treatment
    definition, *xvii*, 90
    discussion of medication regimen
        during psychotherapy session, 25,
        30–31, 35
    effectiveness, 3, 118
    panic disorder, 90–95
    planning, 86
    see also combined treatment;
        psychotherapy with
        pharmacotherapy; sequencing of
        therapies
interpersonal functioning
    bipolar disorder and, 30
    inability to accept nurturance, 20–21
    panic disorder manifestations, 91
    self-other representations, 106–107
interpersonal psychotherapy
    for bipolar disorder, 137
    in combined therapy for depression,
        123, 125–126, 127
    eating disorder treatment, 130
interpersonal social rhythms therapy, 137

Kava Kava, 64
Klonopin. *see* clonazepam

lamotrigine, 120
Learning Psychotherapy, xvii
legal issues in split treatment, 153
limbic system, 163, 174, 175, 178; *see also*
    neurobiology of psychotherapy
lithium, 17–18, 26, 28, 31, 136
lorazepam, 42

malpractice, 36
managed care, 73, 75
    split treatment and, 78, 82, 118, 143,
        154
memory processes
    amygdala in, 165–171
    emotional processing, 165–171
    hippocampal structures in, 162–165
    see also neurobiology of
        psychotherapy
methadone, 131–132
milieu therapy, 133
mind-brain conceptualization, *xv, xvi,*
    10–11, 71
    neurobiology of psychotherapy,
        105–108
mirtazapine, 53
monoamine oxidase inhibitors, 18
monotherapy, 4, 5; *see also*
    pharmacotherapy alone;
    psychotherapy alone
motivational enhancement therapy, 87

naltrexone, 131
Nardil. *see* phenelzine
nefazodone, 5, 125
neurobiology of psychotherapy, 105–108,
    161–162, 178–180
    change processes in, 105, 106–108,
        170–172, 175, 178–179
    circuits model, 105–106
    concept of psychopathology, 105–106,
        107, 162, 167, 168, 169, 172,
        174–177
    dream processes, 177–178
    emotional functioning, 165–171
    implications for treatment, 179–180
    memory processes, 162–165
    models of executive function,
        172–174
    psychoneurosis concept, 162
nonadherence. *see* adherence
noradrenergic system, 167; *see also*
    neurobiology of psychotherapy
nortriptyline, 126

obsessive-compulsive disorder (OCD), 4,
    173–174, 176
    case vignette, 23, 26–27, 29, 31

treatment effectiveness, 6, 129, 138
off-label drug use, 120
olanzapine, 120
oxcarbazepine, 42

panic disorder, *xvi*, 4
    assessment, 89–90
    case vignette, 16–17, 42, 58–59, 62, 68,
        95–103
    neurobiological model, 106, 177
    pharmacotherapy adherence, 44, 45,
        51–52, 63, 65
    phobic stimuli, 89
    treatment algorithm, 90–95
    treatment outcomes, 6, 127–129
    treatment strategies, 88–89
paranoid ideation, 17–18, 28
paroxetine, 17, 47, 49, 63
patient, difficult, 18–19
Paxil. *see* paroxetine
personality disorders, 88
personal therapy, 4, 134
pharmacotherapy. *see* specific drug
pharmacotherapy alone
    inadequacies, 113
    patient choice, 13, 30
    relapse risk, 7
    see also monotherapy
phenelzine, 18–29, 45, 63
phobias, 89
placebo effect, 114–115, 119–120
posttraumatic stress disorder (PTSD),
    xvi, 129–130, 167
prefrontal cortex, 173; *see also*
    neurobiology of psychotherapy
pregnancy, pharmacotherapy and, 41–42,
    62
procedural learning, 107–108
procedural memory, 107
psychoeducational therapy, 136
psychoneurosis, 162
psychopathology
    biopsychosocial model, 121–122
    mind-brain conceptualization, *xv*
    neurobiological model, 105–106, 107,
        162, 167, 168, 174–177
psychotherapy. *see* specific therapy
psychotherapy alone
    contraindications, 132
    inadequacies, 113
    indications, 122
    to prevent relapse after
        pharmacotherapy, 7
    see also monotherapy
psychotherapy with pharmacotherapy
    additive effects in change process,
        113–117

adherence issues, 37, 117
    conceptual basis, *xv–xvi*, 10–11,
        111–118, 178–180
    concerns, 112–113
    effectiveness/efficacy, 111–112
    indications, 4
    matching therapies and drugs, 6–7
    neurobiology, 105–108
    panic disorder treatment strategies,
        88–89
    patient understanding of practice
        standards, 73–74
    personality disorder treatment, 88
    pharmacotherapy goals, 120–121
    phases of pharmacotherapy, 121
    possible negative outcomes, 9–10,
        141–142
    rationale, 112–118
    research needs, 6–7
    research questions, 8–10
    for schizophrenia, 133
    single provider *versus* split treatment,
        10
    social attitudes, 143
    source of prescriptions, 71
    substance abuse treatment, 87–88
    treatment planning, 121–122
    utilization trends, 71
    see also combined treatment;
        integrated treatment; sequencing
        of therapies

raphe nuclei, 106; *see also* neurobiology
    of psychotherapy
referrals
    collegial, 75
    good practice, 74
    obligatory, 75
    perceived by patient as rejection,
        79–80, 83
    sources of, 74–75
relapse, 7, 126–127
Remeron. *see* mirtazapine
research needs, 6–7
    change processes, 108
    combined treatment, 138–139
resistance, *xvii*
risperidone, 28

schizophrenia, 60, 61, 86, 167
    combined treatment, 112–113,
        133–135, 138
    psychopharmacotherapy rationale, 4
    resistance to treatment, 114
selective serotonin reuptake inhibitors
    (SSRI), 6, 88–89, 128–129, 129. see also
    specific drug

self-other representations, 106–107, 108
sequencing of therapies, 116
  case vignette, 95–103
  determinants of, 85
  diagnostic factors in, 86
  panic disorder treatment, 90–95
  research challenges, 85
  strategies, 86–87
  for substance abuse, 87–88; see also
    combined treatment, integrated
    treatment, psychotherapy with
    pharmacotherapy
serotonergic system, 106, 176; see also
  neurobiology of psychotherapy
sertraline, 16–17, 23, 47, 50, 103, 125, 130
Serzone. see nefazodone
sexuality/sexual behavior
  drug side effects, 45, 49, 50, 52–53,
    76–77, 82, 103
  self-value and, 65
side effects, 37, 51–53, 54, 61, 66, 69
  and coherence, 49, 50, 51–53, 54, 61,
    66, 76–77, 82
  clonazepam, 98, 99
  food interactions, 45, 63
  selective serotonin reuptake
    inhibitors, 129
  sexual functioning, 45, 49, 50, 52–53,
    76–77, 82, 103
social anxiety, 4, 122, 130
  case vignette, 16–17, 49
social skills training, 134–135
split treatment, xvii, xix
  benefits, 145–150
  case examples, 141, 144–145
  confidentiality in, 156–157
  countertransference and, 151–152,
    158
  definition, 118, 142
  determinants of, 75
  efficacy/effectiveness, 118–119,
    143–144
  ethical issues, 153–156
  good practice, 156–160
  historical evolution, 143–144
  indications for, 79, 82–83
  legal issues of, 153
  managed care and, 78, 82, 118, 143,
    154
  patient characteristics, 75
  patient understanding of practice
    standards, 73–74
  potential problems of, 141–142,
    150–156
  practice guidelines, 142–143
  relationship between practitioners,
    74–76, 77, 148–149, 150

  single provider versus, 10
  termination, 159
  therapeutic contract in, 76
  therapeutic relationship in, 75, 76,
    147, 151–152
  transference in, 151–152, 158
  treatment design, 74, 157
substance abuse, 50, 60, 68, 70
  adherence issues, 51, 65
  treatment approaches, 87–88
  treatment outcomes, 131–132
supportive-dynamic therapy, 130
supportive psychotherapy, 36, 68, 131

temperament and character, 88
termination, 70–71
  and adherence, 36
  case vignettes, 54–55, 57, 67, 70–71
  in combined therapy, 16
  countertransference issues in, 57, 67,
    70–71
  good practice, 66–67
  grief issues in, 32
  implications for pharmacotherapy, 36
  perceived as abandonment, 83–84
  of pharmacotherapy, 68
  in split treatment, 159
  therapist fears in, 24–25, 30
  therapist guilt in, 22, 29
thalamus, 163; see also neurobiology of
  psychotherapy
therapeutic contract, 76
therapeutic relationship
  adherence to medication regimen
    and, 35–36
  boundary-crossing patient, 81, 83
  culturally sensitive practice, 147–148
  panic disorder treatment, 90
  pharmacotherapy and, 13–15, 28, 36,
    57–58, 67, 112
  in split treatment, 75, 76, 147,
    151–152
  therapist anxiety and, 53, 66
therapist psychotherapy, 32
Thioridazine, 96–97
Tofranil. see imipramine
training and education of
  psychotherapists, xviii, xxi, 144–145
transference, xvi, xvii
  medication adherence and, 45–46, 63
  sexualized, 19
  split treatment and, 151–152, 158
trazodone, 52–53
treatment design
  combined therapy, 14–15

common features of
  psychotherapeutic approaches,
  xvii–xviii
deficit matching, 86–87
determinants of, 86
integrated treatment, 86
neurobiologic considerations,
  179–180
patient role in, 13, 30, 87
psychopharmacotherapy, *xvii,*
  121–122
resource matching, 86, 87
severity matching, 86, 87
split treatment, 74, 157
strategies for, 86–87
see also sequencing of therapies
treatment outcomes
  anxiety disorders, 129–130
  bipolar disorder, 136–138
  combined treatments, 3, 5–6, 112–118
  depression, 123–127
  by diagnosis, 4–6
  eating disorders, 130–131
  integrated treatment, 3
  measurement, 4–5, 113–115

monotherapy, 4–5
new drug development and approval,
  119–120
obsessive-compulsive disorder, 129
panic disorder, 127–129
pharmacotherapy goals, 120–121
possible negative interactions in
  psychopharmacotherapy, 9–10
psychotherapy alone, 122
schizophrenia, 133–135
single provider care *versus* split
  treatment, 118–119
substance abuse, 131–132
tricyclic antidepressants, 124, 125–126.
  see also *specific drug*
Trileptal. *see* oxcarbazepine
twelve-step programs, 87

venlafaxine, 52–53, 57–58, 59, 67
verbal response modes, *xvii*

withdrawal effects, 7

Zoloft. *see* sertraline